When Midwifery Became the Male Physician's Province

To Mike and Miso

EUCHARIUS RÖSSLIN

When Midwifery Became the Male Physician's Province

The Sixteenth Century Handbook
*The Rose Garden for Pregnant Women
and Midwives,* Newly Englished

*Translated from the German and
with an Introduction by*
WENDY ARONS

McFarland & Company, Inc., Publishers
Jefferson, North Carolina, and London

British Library Cataloguing-in-Publication data are available

Library of Congress Cataloguing-in-Publication Data

Rösslin, Eucharius, d. 1526.
    [Swangern Frawen und hebammen Rosegarten. English]
    When midwifery became the male physician's province : the
sixteenth century handbook The rose garden for pregnant women and
midwives / by Eucharius Rösslin ; translated by Wendy Arons. —
Newly Englished.
      p. cm.
    Translation of: Der swangern Frawen und hebammen Rosegarten.
    Includes bibliographical references and index.
    ISBN 0-89950-934-7 (lib. bdg. : 55# alk. paper) ∞
    1. Obstetrics—Early works to 1800. I. Arons, Wendy, 1964– .
II. Title.
RG91.R71513   1994
618.2—dc20   93-42981
                                                      CIP

Manufactured in the United States of America

McFarland & Company, Inc., Publishers
  Box 611, Jefferson, North Carolina 28640

ACKNOWLEDGMENTS

Several people lent crucial assistance to this project both in its initial and final stages. I am very grateful to Ingeborg Glier and James Schultz of the Department of Germanic Languages and Literature at Yale University for their patient assistance and instruction in the translation of sixteenth-century German when I began this project in 1986. Keith Luria of the History Department at Yale was instrumental in shaping and focusing the direction of my initial research. Extra special thanks and eternal gratitude goes to Katrin Sieg, who generously spent many hours helping me work through the more difficult passages of translation and who also provided valuable criticism and suggestions on the introduction. And there are no words to thank Mike Perdriel, without whose loving support and encouragement this project would never have been completed.

TABLE OF CONTENTS

vii

TRANSLATOR'S INTRODUCTION

With the publication of *Der Swangern frawen und he bammen roszgarten* ("The Rose Garden for Pregnant Women and Midwives") at the beginning of the sixteenth century Eucharius Rösslin earned the title of "Europe's Midwives' Teacher" and ended a 1,400-year hiatus in medical literature on pregnancy and childbirth. One of the earliest handbooks for midwives published in a vernacular language, *Roszgarten* (hereinafter referred to as the movie modern version *Rosengarten*) was the authority on midwifery throughout Europe for nearly 200 years. It is frequently cited as a milestone on the road to the professionalization of obstetrics and gynecology by traditional and feminist historians alike (in, respectively, positive and negative contexts). Yet this designation is somewhat problematic. Written by a man who had never attended a delivery and who was dependent on ancient sources for his information, the book did not necessarily reflect the actual practice of midwifery at the time, and whether it led to an improvement in midwifery is a matter of historic debate. The primary manner in which it was a milestone is that it marked the beginning of an encroachment into the midwives' domain by the male medical profession. As the first and by far the most influential text on midwifery of the early modern period, *Rosengarten* is a locus in which the competing forces which shaped the history of midwifery are revealed.

About the Author and the Book

Eucharius Rösslin was born toward the end of the fifteenth century in either modern Oberbaden or Swabia. He lived in

1

Freiburg from about 1493 until 1506. On September 5, 1506, he was engaged as the city physician in Frankfurt am Main at a salary of 60 florins per year for six years. In 1508 he was invited to serve for a short while as physician at the court of Duchess Katherine of Brunswick and Lüneburg, to whom he dedicated *Rosengarten*. He left his position in Frankfurt in 1511 to become city physician in Worms. In 1517 he return to his former position in Frankfurt at a slightly higher salary, and he remained there until his death in 1526. Very little else about Rösslin is known. He was trained as an apothecary and is mentioned as "Apotheker" in 1493 and 1498 in the Register of Guilds of Freiburg.[1] There is no record of Rösslin's attending a university, but his biographer, Karl Baas, finds evidence that he was associated with a university in 1504 when he resided in Freiburg, leading to the presumption that he attended that city's famous university. Rösslin's knowledge of the ancient texts and his reference to his "medical education" in the dedication to *Rosengarten* also suggest that he attended university; it is, moreover, unlikely that he would have been engaged as a city physician without university credentials.[2] As city physician, Rösslin was in charge of all aspects of public health, including coordinating health care in times of plague and epidemic, overseeing and certifying the city's apothecaries, and giving his medical opinion before the council or court when necessary. He was also responsible for the examination and licensing of potential midwives.[3]

Rösslin wrote *The Rose Garden for Pregnant Women and Midwives* in 1513, during his tenure as city physician of Worms. It was, to judge from its publishing history, an immensely popular book. It was reprinted 14 times between 1513 and 1541 under the same title, and 10 times in an expanded edition between 1562 and 1608 under the title *Hebammenbüchlein (Midwives' Booklet)*. In 1532 Rösslin's son, also Eucharius, translated the book into Latin and published it under the title *De Partu Hominis*. From Latin it was further translated into Dutch (28 editions), French (first edition appearing in 1536), Spanish, Danish, Czech, and English. The English edition, entitled *The Byrth of Mankynde*, was translated by Richard Jonas in 1540 and contained the first English copper-plate engravings.[4] Widely disseminated throughout Europe, *Rosengarten* remained the standard handbook on midwifery throughout the sixteenth and well into the seventeenth century.[5]

The immediate popularity of *Rosengarten* indicates that it filled a definite need within the community of midwives. This is due primarily to the dearth of printed information available on midwifery at the time. Prior to the publication of *Rosengarten,* the bulk of material on women's health issues had been written in Latin, a language in which women were largely illiterate. Two important books in the vernacular on women's health preceded *Rosengarten,* Ortolff von Bayerland's *Das Frauen Büchlein* (1500) and "The English Trotula Manuscript" (early fifteenth century).[6] The first was chiefly a collection of dietary guidelines, medications, salves, and ointments for women and did not concern itself with midwifery. The second was a translation of Trotula's *Diseases of Women* of the eleventh century, and although it did contain information on childbirth and pregnancy, it was a manuscript and never received wide distribution.[7] More comprehensive than either of its predecessors, *Rosengarten* was the first vernacular handbook to focus solely on pregnancy, childbirth, and the duties of the midwife.

Technical factors also contributed to its popularity. *Rosengarten* benefited heavily from the technology of the printing press, which made a large distribution possible, and also from the enthusiasm of its publisher, who recognized its commercial potential.[8] Its large readership was also attributable in part to the educational reforms of the Protestant Reformation, which brought about a rise in literacy among the general population of Germany (men and women alike).[9] Particularly noteworthy here is evidence that midwives were expected to be able to read: in her case study of early modern midwifery, Merry Wiesner notes that midwives in Nuremberg "were given printed copies of their oath and of baptism regulations so that they would be able to refer to them if questions arose; no provision was made to have these read to midwives who were illiterate."[10] In addition, later in the century many German cities began to require the midwife to possess a handbook before she could be licensed: this undoubtedly helped to increase the distribution of *Rosengarten*.[11]

But even though its popularity indicates a relatively large interest in and readership for the book, it is debatable whether or not *Rosengarten* reflected the contemporary practice of midwives. The sources for Rösslin's information, as he indicates in his prologue, were the "highly learned skillful scientists/ Galen/ Rhazes/ Avicenna/ Averroes and others." Among these "others" were Hippocrates, Vincent of Beauvais, Guy de Chauliac, Franz von Piemont, Savonarola, and, most importantly, Soranus.[12] The majority of information in *Rosengarten* has been traced back to Soranus's *Gynecology* of 100 A.D.; Rösslin appears to have had access to it in a translation by Muscio from the ninth century. The illustrations which accompany the text were also copied from Muscio's manuscript. In other words, the information in *Rosengarten* predated its appearance by over 1,400 years. Despite the relative stagnation which marked most fields (particularly medicine) during the Middle Ages, it is highly unlikely that the art of midwifery remained virtually unchanged for nearly 14 centuries. A few feminist historians, in fact, maintain the opposite. Ricarda Scherzer claims that midwifery was a highly developed profession in the medieval period, and that the midwife's knowledge was based not only upon personal experience but also on observations built up over generations, and Merry Wiesner points to evidence that midwives were highly valued for their knowledge and skill.[13] This contradicts the analysis of many historians, who take Rösslin at his word when he writes in his prologue of "the midwives each and all / Who know so little of their call / That through neglect and oversight / They destroy children far and wide." Basing their interpretations on Rösslin's condemnation of midwives, these historians maintain that midwifery had deteriorated greatly in the medieval period, and began to advance again only after the publication of *Rosengarten*.[14] To a certain extent, the question of the quality of midwifery before the publication of *Rosengarten* is open to interpretation, since there are very few records left behind by midwives themselves. But to judge the quality of the midwives' work from books written by medical men is risky, because the early modern period was the beginning of a time of professional tension between midwives and medical men, and this tension (and not their ineptitude) may be the reason why midwives were so heavily criticized.

Thus the question of whether *Rosengarten* is a record of the actual practice of midwifery at the time it was written is important not only in terms of medical history but also in terms of the social context in which it appeared. If, as feminist historians now maintain, midwives had indeed improved their profession in the 1,400 years between Soranus and Rösslin, then *Rosengarten* represents a step backward for the art of midwifery, and its authoritative influence must be explained by factors other than its supposed technological superiority or innovation. Perhaps chief among these was the sheer power behind the written word, which effectively conferred upon *Rosengarten* the status of truth. The fact that Rösslin had a position of prestige and power lent additional weight to his word, regardless of his lack of expertise and experience. But above all, *Rosengarten* appeared at the same time as and was part of a general effort to regulate midwives and bring them under the purview of the state apparatus. Viewed in its historical context, *Rosengarten* reveals as much (if not more) about the changing status of midwives in the sixteenth century as it does about the practice of midwifery at the time.

Historical Context to Rosengarten

Not much is known about midwifery in Germany during the medieval period. Using medieval literary texts as her source, Scherzer maintains that midwives had a practice rich in skill and tradition. They had extensive knowledge of herbal remedies for easing pains and releasing cramps, and they recognized the importance of keeping a premature baby warm (as early as the ninth century a premature infant was placed in the hide of a freshly slaughtered pig to keep it warm).[15] Descriptions of the birth of Jesus from the Middle Ages show both the medieval understanding of the necessity of the midwife at a birth and also some of her diagnostic and curative skills. According to legends which date from the ninth century, Joseph went searching for a midwife as the delivery neared and met Zelemi and Salome. These two, upon hearing of the virgin conception, went to verify it for themselves. When they arrived at the manger, Mary had just delivered. The two midwives first took care of the baby, and then manually examined Mary, who, to their astonishment, proved to be a virgin. That these two had experience in midwifery is evident from a twelfth-century version of this legend by Werner von Tegernsee. There we learn that the two women had been at childbirths often, and that among their duties were bathing the newborn and removing the afterbirth from the mother.[16] Scherzer concludes from this and other evidence that even though the medieval midwife did not receive a formal, scientific education, she was well versed in her art. She learned from experience and through an informal apprenticeship system which passed information down through generations.

Beginning in the late Middle Ages, midwives found themselves increasingly the subject of interest from church and government authorities. The original impulse for regulating midwives grew not out of a concern about their competence but rather in response to the problem of children dying unbaptized. In 1277 the Trier Synod ordered that lay midwives be instructed in emergency baptism in case the priest was unable to reach the newborn before it died, and in many cities the thirteenth-century midwife was duty bound by the church to remove a child from its dead mother by Caesarean section in order to prevent its unbaptized death.[17] These early church ordinances were then followed in the fifteenth and sixteenth centuries by city ordinances, which at first were more concerned with the midwife's ethical behavior than her medical capabilities. The earliest midwives' ordinance was the Regensburg Oath of 1452.

It required midwives to swear to deliver all women, rich or poor; to report illegitimate births to the local authorities; not to drink excessively; and not to leave a poor woman in labor to go to a rich one.[18]

The Ulm Ordinance of 1491 mirrors these four basic provisions and takes a step toward establishing city control over the midwife: it invalidated the former agreement *(Vereinbarung)* under which midwives regulated their profession and provided instead that "no midwife will be accepted before she has been recognized by the sworn doctors as sufficiently educated and practiced."[19] Later ordinances placed restrictions upon the midwife's practice, requiring her to call in a doctor or a more experienced midwife in dangerous cases, discover the name of the father of an illegitimate baby, and swear not to aid in abortion.[20] Significantly, the Passau Ordinance of the late sixteenth century required a degree of literacy in midwives in addition to experience in the field, and in 1557 Freiburg required all midwives to possess a handbook. These and similar provisions suggest the increased use of texts like *Rosengarten* as a supplement to the instruction of midwives.[21] As a city physician, Rösslin was intimately connected to this governmental intervention in the practice of midwifery: not only was he responsible for examining and regulating the city's midwives, but he wrote *Rosengarten* upon the request of a ruler (Duchess Katherine), and it was intended as a tool to be used in standardizing the profession.

To view the governmental interest in midwifery as malicious, however, is a misuse of historic hindsight. The city ordinances, issued and reissued over centuries, did eventually virtually regulate midwives out of business. But the original intent of the ordinances was to set standards for the profession and encourage women to enter the field. In fact, the first ordinances were in part initiated by the midwives, who hoped thus to protect both their class interests and their craft from neglect and deterioration.[22] The ordinances were designed to increase the number of qualified midwives in the city and to establish a system for both education and oversight of the city's midwives.

To make a job more desirable to women, most city ordinances provided a scale of wages for the midwife, and often midwives received special compensation in the form of grain or wood or tax abatements for excellent service.[23] City councils also tried to formalize the education of new midwives by requiring midwives to take on apprentices, whose training period lasted anywhere from one to five years. Wiesner notes that "cities . . . encouraged midwives to take on apprentices so as to make sure there would always be an adequate supply. They did this by pleading and threatening and also, more effectively no doubt, by offering financial rewards. . . . Women often responded by taking on their own daughters as apprentices. . . . This is but one example of a mother handing down an occupation to her daughter in the same way a father would to his son."[24] The education and quality of midwives was overseen by the city's "honorable women" *(Ehrbare Frauen)*, who supervised the midwives, assigned them to indigent mothers, disciplined midwives who did not live up to their oath, and sometimes assisted the city physician in examining the midwife for licensing.[25] Wiesner's research reveals the level of experience and knowledge the midwife was expected to have through the examination questions specified in the Memmingen Ordinance of 1578. To quote but a few: "What food, drink, and baths will help a woman have an easy birth? How does she know if a woman is pregnant and does not simply have some other kind of swelling? . . . How does she know whether the fetus is healthy or sick, dead or alive? What is the normal position for birth, and how is this to be brought about in the case of abnormal presentation? What should be done with the umbilical cord and afterbirth, especially to make sure all of the latter has emerged?"[26]

In contradiction to Rösslin's assessment of the situation, midwives seem to have achieved a level of skill and ability that was highly valued by the city councils. Midwives were rarely allowed to leave the city, except in cases where a woman of high position desired the services of a particular midwife — and even then city officials often refused the request.[27] Some midwives' reputations brought them demands for service from high nobility: in 1439 the queen of Hungary requested a German midwife, and in 1501 Prince Frederick of Brandenburg asked the city of Ulm to send a particular midwife named Schrag. A few midwives were even granted nobility in recognition of their knowledge and service.[28] Midwives had other duties within the city as well: they were often called upon to assist in times of plague and other epidemics and were used by physicians to do vaginal examinations of female patients.[29] Further testimony to their skills lies in the fact that during the early modern period in Germany there were very few complaints recorded against midwives for negligence or malpractice.[30] In assessing the skills of early modern midwives, Wiesner concludes, "They knew as much about the mysteries of birth as contemporary university-trained physicians, or more, and appear to have done their job well. Later judgments of midwives as bungling, slovenly, super-stitious, and inept were not shared by early modern political leaders, for they would not have been so concerned with mak-ing sure enough midwives were available had they held such views."[31]

The flip side of the cities' esteem for the midwife, however, was an increasing control and restriction over her activities which was not always benevolent to her interests. As the or-dinances became more and more restrictive, midwives increas-ingly viewed them as a threat to their livelihood and began to show some resistance to this encroachment on their activities.[32] Up until the promulgation of the city ordinances, midwives had had a monopoly on women's health: men were forbidden access to the lying-in chamber, and it was considered improper and immoral for male doctors to examine women's intimate parts.[33] With the ordinances, midwives were increasingly required to share their exclusive experiential knowledge of childbirth with the male city physician as part of their examination. Midwives often balked at this and refused to give their secrets to the "com-petition."[34]

The midwives' resistance to attempts to coopt their knowledge made it nearly impossible for medical men to learn anything of childbirth outside of the ancient texts, and, as a result, the city physician responsible for examining midwives may have inadvertently lowered the standards for the practice of midwifery out of ignorance of the actual practice. Rösslin's text appears to be an example of this: its dependence on ancient medical texts may have contributed to a later decline in midwifery due to the omission of much information that had earlier been part of the midwife's field of knowledge. In addition, some of the restrictions placed on the midwife removed certain activities and procedures from her area of expertise. For example, the requirement to call in a doctor in difficult cases narrowed the midwife's range of experience and diminished her ability to deal with such cases on her own; likewise with regulations which forbade the use of surgeon's tools or the mixing of drugs.[35] Such provisions were designed more to protect the economic interests of the doctors, barber-surgeons, and apothecaries than the health interests of pregnant women. But these regulations did more than just limit the activities of midwives: they also allowed men to establish an (albeit rather precarious) foothold in an area of medicine which had been up until that time controlled and practiced exclusively by women.

As a result, the regulations concerning midwives which appeared in the fifteenth and sixteenth century mark the slow beginning of what many feminist historians have dubbed a "male takeover of midwifery." Although in Germany male accoucheurs did not gain entry into the delivery room until the eighteenth century, the process toward a masculinization of midwifery (and the later establishment of the medical field of obstetrics and gynecology) was set in motion in the early modern period.

The "takeover" of the profession of midwifery has been analyzed in depth in several recent works, including *Midwives and Medical Men* by Jean Donnison, *Women and Men Midwives* by Jane Donegan, and *Hebammen* by Scherzer, and is beyond the scope of this essay.

The critical methodology behind the idea of a male takeover of midwifery is worth commenting on, however, because it has a direct bearing on any interpretation of *Rosengarten*. This methodology tends to place the transition from the midwife to the medical man in the context of a co-optation of the power of women to control their own health issues. In many ways this is a sound and accurate analysis, in particular when the early modern German midwife's resistance to the encroachment upon her field is taken into account. But there is another side to the issue which is equally critical. Although there is no denying that midwives were edged out of the field of women's health care by medical men, it is a bit romantic to assign to the early modern midwife a position of power, even if she did have primary control over women's health issues. For, as Helen Callaway points out, "childbirth takes place within a male-dominated cultural system which considers female sexuality to be inherently dangerous and controls it through strong ritual restrictions."[36]

That childbirth was managed exclusively by females was originally the result of religious and social taboos which rarely worked to the advantage of women. In sixteenth-century Germany these taboos were based upon "propriety" as defined by the church: men were not allowed into the delivery room because it was considered "improper" for a man to witness a woman in labor.

Consequently, *men* declared midwifery off-limits to themselves, and even though women had control over women's health, they still operated within and under the control of the dominant power structure. The reason this is important to *Rosengarten* is that the fact that this book had such an immediate and profound influence indicates the extent to which midwives were subject to the dominant power structure; a male-dominated world which, because it placed a greater value on the canon of medical literature than it did on the experience of midwives, unquestioningly accepted the validity of a handbook written by a man who had never delivered a child and readily asserted the superiority of his knowledge over that of the midwife. Framed in this context, Rösslin's derogatory comments about midwives in the dedication and prologue to his handbook beg for a new interpretation.

The Dedication and Prologue to Rosengarten

Rosengarten opens with a dedication to Duchess Katherine of Brunswick and Lüneburg, which contains a five-page poem in rhymed couplet entitled "Admonition to Pregnant Women and Midwives." This is followed by a short Prologue in which Rösslin lists the sources for his handbook. Both crucially important parts of the handbook, historians have paid scant attention to these two texts. When they do, they often use Rösslin's remarks against midwives in his prologue to show that the early modern midwife was ignorant and inept. It is precarious, however, to take Rösslin at his word when he castigates midwives, for the primary purpose of both these texts was to establish his authority to write a handbook on midwifery. To this end, he launches a two-pronged attack: he traces his knowledge back to God as its original source, and he simultaneously undermines the authority of the midwife by assailing her abilities.

Rösslin is very careful in the dedication and prologue to leave the reader with no doubts about his qualifications for writing this book. In the first line of the dedication he immediately derives authority from two sources: from the Duchess Katherine, who personally requested him to write the book, and from his status as a doctor. He mentions his profession five times within the first 12 pages of the book, a gesture designed not only to confer upon himself the prestige of the university but also to elevate himself above the average midwife, who may have had more practical knowledge of parturition but who was denied access to universities and the classical texts they taught.

He then proceeds to legitimate his handbook through a series of references to God. The first comes in the dedication, where he relates the story of Eve:

> I find in the third chapter of the book of creation/ That the almighty eternal God/ punished our very first mother Eve/ for violating the commandment/ with the curse/ that she should bear her children in pain/ This curse is inherited from her by all women/ and although this pain may not be completely

abolished or hindered by any reason/ wisdom/ or art/ yet if pregnant women prepare and behave themselves properly before and during the delivery/ and take precautions with wise learned women and midwives/ then such pain may be tempered and lessened.

This book, he continues, contains "everything that it is necessary for the pregnant bearing woman and midwife to know." The implication is clear: although God's curse on womankind is an inevitable evil, Rösslin assumes for himself the power and authority to tell midwives and women how to alleviate the pain associated with God's will.

The Admonition which follows the dedication continues in this vein. It contains numerous references to God which link God's benevolence toward mankind with Rösslin's service to the female community in publishing *Rosengarten*. The poem begins by associating the power of God and the power of a father. Rösslin writes that God redeemed mankind with his own blood "as any father's done / Who tears apart both body and land / At seeing his child in danger's hands." Even though this is a book for mothers, Rösslin puts father and God in the enviable position of being the ones who can save a child—just as, presumably, the male doctor should when called in by the midwife, or as Rösslin claims to do with this book. Rösslin later associates himself with God's interests by describing how it hurts them both to see a soul lost. He then invokes God's anger as a threat to the midwife who does not do her job properly—that is, according to *Rosengarten*. The poem ends with the hope that even if Rösslin earns nothing from the book in this life, God will reward him in the next.

Rösslin's ultimate association of himself with God, however, comes in the Prologue, where he traces the knowledge in the book directly from God. He describes how God made man from nothing and gave him the treasure of his wisdom, which was passed down through the "highly learned skillful scientists/ Galen/ Rhazes/ Avicenna/ Averroes and others whom it is not necessary to name" to Rösslin himself. Rösslin thus establishes himself as the ultimate recipient of the divine knowledge of midwifery, a knowledge which is by definition infinite and all-encompassing. With this, he gives the information in the handbook legitimacy and himself impeccable credentials.

This strategy of legitimation was a common feature of prologues to nonfictive German literature of the medieval period. In her study of the prologue, Helga Unger notes that authors used the prologue to prove both the correctness of the facts and the authenticity of the mediator. "The truth and dignity of the subject matter was central. It was attempted to 'prove' this through an invocation of God himself as the original author and guarantor, usually in connection with references to a (written) source."[37] But, given the context in which Rösslin wrote *Rosengarten* and the audience for which it was intended, such legitimation takes on additional meaning. Rösslin had no experience in midwifery, a circumstance which, given the ban on men in the delivery room, would have been self-evident to his contemporaries. The prologue thus responds to a very real need to justify his writing. More importantly, his invectives against midwives are tossed under the same blanket of authority and truth used to legitimate the content of the handbook. *Rosengarten* was not only a book for midwives; it was also written for pregnant women, who were accustomed to entrusting their medical care to midwives. In the dedication and prologue he establishes his authority and then authoritatively undermines the midwife, thereby sowing the seeds of mistrust and creating an audience among pregnant women receptive both to his book and to the entrance of men into the field of midwifery.

Considering the midwives' resistance to encroachment upon their profession by medical men, Rösslin's criticism of them is often heavy with double meaning. In the Admonition Rösslin claims that "since no midwife that I've asked / Could tell me anything of her task / I'm left to my medical education / Which takes such things in consideration." He uses the implication of midwives' ignorance as justification for presenting the works of Soranus and others as an improvement on midwifery of the day. But, given the tension between midwives and medical men, it is just as likely that the midwife *could* tell him something of her task but *wouldn't*. Rösslin's accusations against the midwives of ignorance, murder, negligence, and careless-ness should be similarly scrutinized. He charges, among other things, that midwives "take life while doing their duty," kill "by . . . dumb mismanagement," and take away eternal life. But these accusations have little basis in fact, and appear to be almost solely politically motivated. In attacking the character and reputation of his opponent, Rösslin chose a highly effective tactic for establishing authority and expertise in a field in which he had neither. He was so masterful at it, in fact, that historians have taken him at his word for centuries.[38] But although there undoubtedly were many inept midwives at this time, it seems more instructive to read Rösslin's denigration of midwives as an indication of the circumstances surrounding his writing rather than as a true description of the state of the midwifery.

Aside from painting a rather exaggerated picture of the dire straits of midwifery, some of Rösslin's criticism also in-directly associates the midwife with witchcraft. He claims that "one finds such evil women / Who give to death a cause and reason / That the fruit from life is driven." The word "fruit" ("frucht") is tantalizingly ambiguous — it could mean an early fetus or a fully developed infant — and allows for a variety of in-terpretations. Rösslin may be charging midwives of infanticide, abortion, or providing birth control — all of which were asso-ciated with witchcraft. In the *Malleus Maleficarum (Hammer of Witches)* of 1484 among the evils performed by witches were those of "destroying the generative force in women . . . procur-ing abortion . . . [and] offering children to the devils."[39] The ac-cusation of witchcraft is also implied in the charge that midwives allowed children to die unbaptized. The charge of witchcraft was often a political weapon aimed at women healers whenever their wisdom or healing powers were seen as threat-ening to the church and state. Here the implied warning to the pregnant woman that her midwife might possibly be a witch serves the dual purpose of denigrating the midwife's skills and fostering a general feeling of distrust and suspicion against her.

But for all his claims to authority and legitimation, the work Rösslin produced was not an improvement on the art of midwifery. His reliance on ancient medical texts produced a somewhat confused version of female anatomy and the positions of the fetus in the womb, and he passed along much superstition along with his medical advice. He also curiously omitted a number of rather important bits of information from his sources. Most notable among these is Soranus's warning to the midwife to wash her hands and pare her fingernails before inserting her hand into the uterus—a vital precaution which is nowhere to be found in *Rosengarten*.[40] Rösslin also makes no mention of pica, and only briefly mentions the umbilical cord, subjects which Soranus deals with at some length. Although he gives instructions on how to deal with a torn perineum, he fails to include Soranus's technique for supporting the woman's anus and perineum during delivery—a technique which was in practice among midwives at the time.[41] In addition, his description of a "natural" birth as one in which the baby appears with its face up must have struck the midwife as unusual, since in a normal delivery the baby comes out with its face down. Although some of the advice given in *Rosengarten* is good common sense, most of it was probably quite ineffectual, a problem Rösslin implicitly acknowledges by including a section on how to recognize if the woman is dead and a chapter on removing the dead baby from the womb. Because he had no experience in delivering children to support his selection of information from among the classics, Rösslin's advice was of dubious value to the midwife. And yet, despite the fact that the book might have contradicted the midwife's experience on several points, it was widely accepted and grew to have great influence. Rösslin's call to the authority of the ancients superseded any knowledge based upon experience and observation, and thus much of what was really valuable in medieval and early modern midwifery was lost in deference to Soranus, Hippocrates, Galen, and Avicenna.

Ironically, later writers frequently complained that "meddlesome midwives" endangered the mother because they used the very techniques recommended in *Rosengarten*. It is not known how many of these techniques were part of the midwife's practice before the publication of *Rosengarten,* but it is certain that they became standard once the book was in circulation. Thus, to an extent, *Rosengarten* not only created a receptivity for masculine authority in midwifery; it also played a role in the decline in midwifery which was used in the eighteenth century as a justification for male entry into the field.[42]

The Handbook

The handbook itself consists of 12 chapters, dealing with nearly every aspect of childbirth from prenatal care to the handling of normal and abnormal deliveries to the care of the newborn. It contains several illustrations, most notably the famous "birth figures" showing various positions of the fetus in the womb. It also has a picture of a birth stool and an engraving which depicts Rösslin presenting his book to the Duchess Katherine. The book ends with a table listing the Latin and German names for the herbs mentioned in the body of the text.

Perhaps the most striking feature of the handbook is the series of birth figures. In an article on *Rosengarten* which appeared in the *Journal of Obstetrics and Gynæcology of the British Empire* in 1909, E. Ingerslev traces these illustrations to the Muscio translation of the Soranus manuscript, and shows that they appeared throughout Europe in various manuscripts during the medieval period.[43] These illustrations depict the womb as a sort of inverted flask or balloon with the mouth pointing down; and the babies inside resemble miniature adults with fully grown hair and in a variety of (sometimes quite fantastic) positions. Although in his text Rösslin correctly describes the baby in the womb as "curled and bent like a round ball," the illustrations show the babies with outstretched limbs and upright head. These illustrations appeared in all of the editions of the handbook, including the translations, and were some of the most widely distributed pictures of the early modern period. But they did not reflect a contemporary understanding of anatomy: as early as 1490 Leonardo da Vinci had produced detailed depictions of infants in the womb from dissection, and a slightly more modern text by Jane Sharp contains a more accurate illustration of the baby in the womb.[44]

Also noteworthy are the scores of herbal remedies listed in the book. The early modern midwife needed to have a broad knowledge of herbal preparation and a ready supply available whenever she attended a labor. As an apothecary, Rösslin must have had an extensive knowledge of the properties of herbs, and the recipes he gives were probably a compilation of his own knowledge and lists from his other sources. Similar recipes can be found in Soranus and Avicenna, but not to the extent listed in *Rosengarten*. Many of Rösslin's herbal preparations may have been quite effective: particularly striking is a recipe from Chapter Five for a pain-relieving pill containing "one-fifth of a dram of a juice called opium" which was to be administered with a glass of wine(!).

Some of the treatments he recommends may appear bizarre or dangerous to the modern reader but were quite common medical practice based on the scientific theories of the day. For example, the technique of fumigating the womb with pleasant-smelling substances to draw out the afterbirth or a dead baby is a remedy recommended by Hippocrates in the *Aphorisms,* and although Soranus calls such fumigations "futile," it was a standard technique for many centuries before and after the publication of *Rosengarten.*[45] Cupping and bleeding were common remedies based on the writings of both Hippocrates and Galen, and Rösslin prudently passes along Hippocrates's warnings against the excessive or untimely bleeding of pregnant women.[46] Rösslin also includes a number of beliefs about pregnancy and childbirth which seem superstitious but which were similarly part of the accepted scientific canon. The idea that a boy lay on the right side and a girl on the left and that the corresponding breast shrivels to indicate the death of the baby is Hippocratic, as are most of the descriptions of the causes of miscarriage listed in Chapter Eight.[47] The notion that a baby born in the seventh or ninth month would live, but one born in the eighth month would not comes from Albertus Magnus, who maintained that "the fetus became very active in the seventh month of gestation, that it rested from its exertions in the eighth month and at the end of the ninth month it comes into the world healthy and strong. If, perchance, it was born in the eighth month having been exhausted from its strong movements in the previous month, it would surely die because of fatigue."[48] Numerology was also used to support this theory. Jane Sharp, relying on many of the same sources as Rösslin in her work of 1671, explains that "women are all ready to be brought a bed at seven moneths [sic] end, for that number of seven is the perfection of all numbers."[49] Rösslin also reflects the contemporary theory that a boy was easier to deliver than a girl in his instruction to the midwife to "promise the mother the happy delivery/ of a baby boy."

Included among the plasters, herbs, and fumigations are some treatments and techniques which are surprisingly sophisticated for the day. Although Rösslin generally insists that the best method for dealing with an abnormal delivery is by turning the baby to a head presentation, he hints at the possibility of delivering the baby by the feet, a technique known as "podalic version" and promoted by Ambroise Paré later in the sixteenth century.[50] His suggestion for repairing a torn perineum using plaster instead of sutures is both practical and humane, considering the lack of anesthesia in the early modern period. In addition, his dietary recommendations for nursing and pregnant women read as good common sense, and are especially noteworthy for an age when women rarely received adequate nutrition.[51]

One of the most curious things about the handbook is the apparent contradiction between the book's instructions to midwives and certain legal restrictions on the practices of women healers. As part of an effort to protect the economic interests of apothecaries and barber-surgeons, women healers (and "quacks") were frequently forbidden by law to mix drugs or use surgeon's tools.[52] Yet Rösslin gives detailed instructions to the midwife on both the preparation of herbal medications and the use of tools to extract a dead baby from the womb. He even gives instructions on how to perform a Caesarean section in case of the death of the mother. Wiesner explains this contradiction by noting that the city councils were "willing to let a woman do things they looked upon as an extension of her job as a midwife.... When she was treating pregnant women and infants ... there were no restrictions on what she could do."[53] But there are also other explanations for the inclusion of such methods in *Rosengarten*. Although the city midwife had relatively quick access to a doctor or apothecary in case of emergency, the isolated country midwife was frequently left to her own devices when faced with a difficult delivery. Since it was often impossible for her to get help in time, she needed to know how to perform the tasks of the apothecary and surgeon. In addition, since medical men had no access to the delivery room, these portions of the book may also have been intended to teach them how to proceed when called in by the midwife. Nonetheless, it is highly interesting that the book implicitly acknowledges that, despite the regulations, midwives did perform these activities.

One final comment about *Rosengarten* concerns its unusual title. The use of the image of a rose garden refers on one level to the site where the midwife gathered her medicinal herbs. The book is called *Rosengarten* because it represents a similar compendium of life-saving remedies. But at the end of the Admonition Rösslin offers an expansion of this image:

> And so the name of this book is
>   The pregnant woman's Garden of Roses
> In which you dig and pluck the herbs
>   Which have body, life/ and soul on earth
> Such roses which your hands do take
>   Will come in time before God's face
> Therefore you should take special care
>   Have high regard and be aware
> That the roses you select
>   Are the ones that please God best.

His metaphor uses the image of a rose "which pleases God

best" to represent the child which has been properly brought into the world: that is, not only safely delivered, but also baptized. He identifies his *Rosengarten* with God's garden of "roses," the children God selects to go to heaven, implying that the book will help to supply God with a bountiful bouquet. In addition, the title *Rosengarten* is a play on Rösslin's name, which means "little rose."

One of God's "roses" himself, Rösslin has created his own little garden to ensure a place in heaven for all children. In light of his subject matter — maternity — it seems appropriately, if bitterly ironic that by linking this pun on his name to the use of the rose as a symbol for the pregnant woman's children, Rösslin metaphorically claims for himself the role of both father and gardener in the "field" of parturition. For his little book became the seed of change that eventually brought the male doctor into the delivery room and changed the face — and gender — of women's health care for centuries to come.

A Note on the Translation

In translating *Rosengarten* into modern English, I have endeavored to create a text that was accessible to the modern reader and yet still retained the flavor of a sixteenth-century document. To this end, and at the risk of rendering it slightly awkward, I have chosen to retain the punctuation of the German original. Early modern German used the virgule (/) to break up long sentences, separate lists of items, and divide a sentence into clauses much the same way modern English uses a comma. Rösslin was fond of breaking his sentences up into very small parts, often in a way which made the meaning less rather than more clear. In the translation I have omitted virgules where they become confusing. Commas have also been inserted where necessary to make the English sentence clear. I have also retained Rösslin's paragraph mark (¶), which is generally used to indicate the start of a new sentence.

I have chosen to use syntax and phrasing rather than

vocabulary and orthography to achieve a trace of antiquity in this translation. In order to make the text clear to the modern reader, I have avoided the use of outmoded terms and old-fashioned spelling (such as, for example, the use of the word "flowers" for "menstruation," or the spelling "drachm"). I have left Latin terms and phrases in Latin, with a translation where necessary in the footnotes.

This translation is based on the 1910 reprint of *Der Swangern frawen und he bammen roszgarten,* edited by Gustav Klein.

Wendy Arons
San Diego, CA, 1993

Notes

1. For biographical information on Rösslin see Gustav Klein, *Eucharius Rösslins "Rosengarten,"* p. vi; and Karl Baas, *Eucharius Rösslins Lebensgang,* passim.

2. Manfred Stürzbecher, "The Physici in German-Speaking Countries from the Middle Ages to the Enlightenment," p. 124.

3. Karl Baas, "Dr. Eucharius Rösslin: Arzt zu Worms im 16. Jahrhundert," p. 39; Ulrich Knefelkamp, *Das Gesundheits- und Fürsorgewesen der Stadt Freiburg im Breisgau im Mittelalter,* p. 130; and Stürzbecher, p. 126.

4. Klein, pp. xii–xiv; Audrey Eccles, *Obstetrics and Gynecology in Tudor and Stuart England,* p. 11, gives a date of 1532 for a translation into Latin by Christian Egonolph; Klein, p. vi, maintains that Rösslin's son first translated his work. The majority of scholars agree with Klein. See also Walter Radcliffe, *Milestones in Midwifery,* p. 6; and Irving Cutter and Henry Viets, *A Short History of Midwifery,* p. 5.

5. Eccles, p. 12; and J. H. Aveling, *English Midwives: Their History and Prospects,* p. 122.

6. Beryl Rowland, *Medieval Woman's Guide to Health,* pp. xvi, 18.

7. *The Diseases of Women* was, however, written by a woman, Trotula of Salerno, and represents one of the earliest examples of women's medical writing.

8. E. Ingerslev, "Rösslin's 'Rosengarten': Its Relation to the Past (the Muscio Manuscripts and Soranos), Particularly with Regard to Podalic Version," p. 80.

9. Gerald Strauss, "Techniques of Indoctrination: The German Reformation," p. 104. Strauss claims, "one who has spent much time with the

sources cannot suppress the conclusion that reading was a common rather than an uncommon pursuit for a large number of people in nearly all walks of German society in the sixteenth century." Rolf Engelsing, *Analphabetentum und Lektüre,* pp. 32-41, also cites evidence for increasing literacy in Germany during the 16th century. He states, "Im ganzen aber war im 16. Jahrhundert die Lese- und Schreibfähigkeit im deutschen Sprachraum weit verbreitet" (p. 33).

10. Merry E. Wiesner, "Early Modern Midwifery: A Case Study," p. 31.

11. Knefelkamp, p. 132.

12. The following authors all maintain that *Rosengarten* is primarily based on Soranus: H. Fasbender, *Geschichte der Geburtshülfe,* pp. 115–21; Theodore Cianfrani, *A Short History of Obstetrics and Gynecology,* p. 135; Edwin Jameson, *Gynecology and Obstetrics,* pp. 30, 36; and Paul Diepgen, *Frau und Frauenheilkunde in der Kultur des Mittelalters,* p. 112.

13. Ricarda Scherzer, *Hebammen: Weise Frauen oder Technikerinnen? Zum Wandel eines Berufsbildes,* p. 17; and Merry Wiesner, *Working Women in Renaissance Germany,* p. 57.

14. Jean Donnison, *Midwives and Medical Men: A History of Interprofessional Rivalries and Women's Rights,* p. 8; and Muriel Joy Hughes, *Women Healers in Medieval Life and Literature,* p. 110. See also Cianfrani, p. 125.

15. Scherzer, p. 15.

16. *Ibid.,* pp. 16–17.

17. Edward Shorter, *A History of Women's Bodies,* p. 41; Donnison, p. 3; and Scherzer, pp. 26–31.

18. Shorter, p. 41.

19. Alfons Fischer, *Geschichte des deutschen Gesundheitswesens,* 1:87.

20. *Ibid.,* 1:88; Knefelkamp, pp. 130–31; and Wiesner (1986), p. 61.

21. Fischer, p. 89; and Knefelkamp, p. 132. Later, the basis for midwives' examinations in Zurich was Jacob Rueff's *Hebammenbuch,* which was quite similar to *Rosengarten.* See Radcliffe, p. 9; and Harvey Graham, *Eternal Eve,* pp. 147–48.

22. Scherzer, p. 41.

23. Knefelkamp, p. 131.

24. Wiesner (1986), p. 57.

25. *Ibid.,* p. 56.

26. *Ibid.,* p. 62.

27. *Ibid.,* p. 57.

28. Scherzer, p. 49.

29. Wiesner (1986), p. 69; and Jameson, p. 224.

30. Wiesner (1986), pp. 68–69.

31. *Ibid.,* p. 69.

32. Scherzer, p. 48. Cianfrani also refers to midwives' resistance, albeit in a negative way: "In the early Renaissance, when all forms of medicine showed hopeful signs of advance, obstetrics stood still . . . we see belligerent midwives guarding the lying-in chamber against all medical interference, particularly the male species" (p. 125).

33. Jane Donegan, *Women and Men Midwives,* pp. 18-19; Donnison, pp. 11, 55; and Cianfrani, p. 125.

34. Scherzer, pp. 45–46.

35. *Ibid.*, pp. 54, 61.

36. Helen Callaway, "'The Most Essentially Female Function of All': Giving Birth," p. 178. See also Shorter, p. 68; and Ivan Illich, *Gender*, pp. 123–26, for analyses along similar lines.

37. "Meist steht die Wahrheit und Dignität der Sache in Mittelpunkt. Sie wird zur 'beweisen' versucht durch Berufung auf Gott selbst als letzten Urheber und Garanten, meist in Verbindung mit dem Hinweis auf eine (schriftliche) Quelle." Helga Ungar, "Vorreden deutscher Sachliteratur des Mittelalters als Ausdruck literarischen Bewußtseins," p. 250.

38. See Donnison, p. 8; Hughes, p. 110; and Cianfrani, p. 125. Cianfrani and Fasbender testify to Rösslin's "authority," even while admitting the lack of scientific or historic basis to his writing. Fasbender claims, "Man hat nicht mit Unrecht gesagt, daß Roesslin, obgleich selbst nicht ausübender Geburtshelfer, eine Zeitlang der Hebammenlehrer Europas gewesen [war]," p. 121. Cianfrani, on p. 135, states: "*[Rosengarten]* was more widely translated and distributed than any other medical book up to that time, it had no scientific merit, and yet, with its numerous translations it became not only a text book for midwives, but for two centuries served as an authoritative treatise on obstetrics for the medical profession in England and throughout all Europe."

39. Cited in Barbara Ehrenreich and Deirdre English, *Witches, Midwives and Nurses: A History of Women Healers*, p. 11.

40. Soranus, *Soranus' Gynecology*, translated by Owsei Temkin, pp. 72–73, 186–87.

41. *Ibid.*, p. 74. Scherzer, p. 52, gives an example of a handwritten account of this technique.

42. Eccles, pp. 87–89, makes this argument with regards to the publication of *The Byrth of Mankynde* in England. She notes, "[Jonas'] advice . . . in some respects seems to have contributed to a fall in the standards of midwifery during the next hundred years. Much of this advice, and still more the ignorant and over-zealous application of it, was gradually rejected by the writers on midwifery of the next century" (p. 87).

43. Ingerslev, pp. 23–25.

44. Joseph Needham, *A History of Embryology*, p. 96; and Jane Sharp, *The Midwives Book*, pp. 151, 199.

45. Hippocrates, *The Aphorisms of Hippocrates*, translated by Elias Marks, section 5, no. 28; and Soranus, pp. 152–53, 196–98.

46. Hippocrates, 5, no. 50; and Peter Brain, *Galen on Bloodletting*, p. 83.

47. Hippocrates 5, nos. 38, 48; descriptions of miscarriage run throughout section 5.

48. Quoted in Cianfrani, p. 105.

49. Sharp, pp. 173–74.

50. Medical historians are in some disagreement whether to credit Rösslin or Ambroise Paré (1510–90) with the reintroduction of this method, which was used by the ancients, but forgotten or discarded during the medieval period. Since Rösslin heavily favors the head delivery and only briefly suggests the possibility of a foot delivery, Paré is usually credited with rediscovering podalic version. See Ingerslev, pp. 88–90; and Donnison,

pp. 10–11. It is tempting to speculate whether or not this technique was truly "lost" to midwives, or only to the writings of medical men; Ingerslev suggests "the possibility of a tradition (as already hinted by Paré) having preserved a practice which had not found a place in the books" (p. 90).

51. Shorter, p. 51ff.
52. Wiesner (1986), p. 53.
53. *Ibid.,* p. 54.

Der Schwanngeren
frawen vnd Hebam
men Rosengarte.

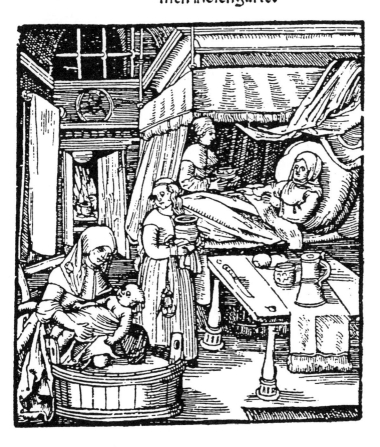

License

We, Maximilian, chosen Emperor of Rome by the grace of God/ at all times Lord of the empires of Germany/ Hungary/ Dalmatia/ Croatia &c. King/ Archduke of Austria/ Duke of Burgundy/ Brabant/ and Pfalzgraf &c. Let it be known that, as our and the empire's honorable beloved loyal Eucharius Rösslin doctor of medicine/ has made various tractat and books for the common use/ and particularly for the furtherance and good of pregnant women and their newborn children/ and is prepared to have them printed and distributed/ We have therefore done and given him this particular honor and license/ and do and give it him here deliberately by the power of this letter/ That no one irrespective of their office/ status/ or character/ may reprint this same book for six years after the date which follows this imperial letter. And if it should be printed outside of the Holy Empire and in foreign nations/ in German or other tongues/ These should not be offered/ sold/ or distributed in the Holy Empire. And in addition with this letter we solemnly summon each and every Elector/ Prince/ spiritual and lay Prelate/ Count/ Freeman/ Lord/ Knight/ Vassal*/ Captain/ Governor/ Bailiff/ Advocate/ Administrator/ Official/ Village Mayor/ City Mayor/ Judge/ Council member/ Citizen/ Commoner/ And all others of our and the Empire's subjects and faithful followers/ irrespective of their office/ status/ or character/ and desire them by dint of this license/ to esteem/ preserve/ and protect the named doctor Eucharius/ And not print/ offer/ or let the above-mentioned books be sold/ And we order that this be honored everywhere in their principalities/ lands/ cities/ dominions/ and

---

*Knecht: *also "journeyman; master-in-training" (Wiesner [1986], pp. 34, 193).*

territories/ That as loved as each may be he may avoid our and the Empire's grave disfavor and punishment/ and also a penalty/ Namely ten marks of pure gold/ which any who so against our license prints/ offers/ or sells these books will forfeit each time such occurs, half to us in our treasury/ and the other half to be paid unconditionally to the named doctor Eucharius/ documented in this letter given in our and the Holy Empire's city of Cologne on the twenty-fourth day of the month of September/ in the fifteen hundred and twelfth year after the birth of Christi/ the twenty-seventh year of our Roman Empire and the twenty-third year of the Hungarian.

Per regem	Ad mandatum domini Im-
per se	peratoris proprium

Sernnteiner.

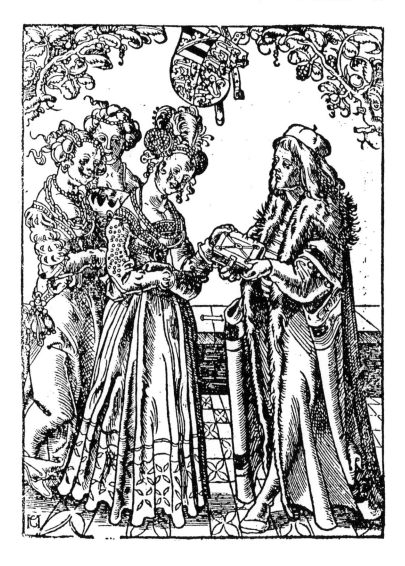

To the illustrious highborn princess and lady/ Lady Katherine born of Saxony/ Duchess of Brunswick and Lüneburg/ to my gracious lady/ I Eucharius Rösslin doctor of medicine/ Offer my humble obedient willing service/ Gracious princess/ I find in the third chapter of the book of creation/ That the almighty eternal God/ punished our very first mother Eve/ for violating the commandment/ with the curse/ that she should bear her children in pain/ This curse is inherited from her by all women/ and although this pain may not be completely abolished or hindered by any reason/ wisdom/ or art/ yet if pregnant women prepare and behave themselves properly before and during the birth/ and take precautions with wise learned women and midwives/ then such pain may be tempered and lessened. Therefore gracious lady/ since Y.R.H.* bade Me several years ago/ to publish learning and instruction for the benefit of pregnant women and midwives/ I am ready and willing out of humble and obedient duty to Y.R.H./ to publish everything that it is necessary for the pregnant bearing woman and midwife to know/ from the most learned doctoribus/ who have written and studied before me. Although Y.R.H. is graced with such reason and knowledge/ that Y.R.H. has no need to be instructed in this and many other things/ There are still many honorable younger women and midwives who have little instruction/ and to whom the knowledge which is collected in this book has been unknown/ for those women this knowledge will be necessary. This therefore is my most humble request of Y.R.H. That Y.R.H. would graciously receive from me this book (called the Rose Garden for Pregnant Women and Midwives)/ and distribute it in Your Highness's Principality/ and in other German lands/ among the honorable modest pregnant women and midwives/ I am of the certain hope that they will find in it adequate instruction on how they should behave themselves in all things. And if Y.R.H. desires to know more instruction/ which is not collected in this book, since not all things are proper to write I am completely willing out of humble

*Your Royal Highness. *The German reads U.F.G. for "Uwer Fürstlichen Gnaden."*

obedient duty to give Y.R.H. oral instruction/ and with this I humbly put myself under the surety and protection of Y.R.H. against calumny and libel. Datum at Worms on the xx. day of the month of February. In the year as counted from the birth of Christi/ fifteen hundred and thirteen.

Admonition to Pregnant Women and Midwives

How very close to man God is
    Each person can deduct from this
That down from heaven's throne came he
    To walk this earthly misery
His creation's comfort to obtain
    And this he earned with such great pain
That he redeemed it with his own
    blood/ as any father's done
Who tears apart both body and land
    At seeing his child in danger's hands
And simple it is to understand
    God's reasons for the work at hand
For he takes care of that soul best
    Which he made in his own likeness
But now it is our shameful plight
    That we cherish a soul so slight
And are not able to perceive
    That it's a noble thing indeed
Whoe'er preserves a soul on earth
    Performs a deed of such great worth
That he receives from God a crown
    And in heaven great renown
In thought and feeling I contend
    That we must work without an end
Whene'er a newborn's brought to light
    To save its soul with all our might
If the body's matter is strong and fit
    And there's no lack of life in it
Then God grants it the noblest life
    And gives a soul to it by and by

I hold this a great gift to be
>For which forever praised be he
Now often we're so ill-prepared
>For what God gives us with such care
That we destroy it totally
>And such great things go unperceived
I mean the midwives each and all
>Who know so little of their call
That through neglect and oversight
>They destroy children far and wide
And work such evil industry
>That they take life while doing their duty
>And earn from this a handsome fee.
If the mother herself did such a deed
>We'd bury her with lightning speed
Alive/ and such an injury
>Is punished on the wheel by imperial decree
If unpunishèd we let her free
>She'll earn from God her penalty
For when a child of life's deprived
>And without holy baptism dies
The guilt is on the midwife's hands
>E'er far from God's countenance must she stand
As God himself shuts heaven's gates
>For she can never atone for the babe
The onus for whose death was hers
>And she cannot this deed reverse
To bring to grace the innocent
>Killed by her dumb mismanagement
We are the ones/ in a few words
>Who are born to live on earth
Whom God gifts with eternal life
>After this troubled time of strife
And are born heaven's citizens
>Hereafter to be chosen ones
Thus each some assistance should give
>That they might help a child to live
Midwives I mean especially
>Who should be trained for their duty
So that they earn their salary

Just when they do things properly
Now there is so much negligence
    That it lies on my conscience
And much it pains me in my heart
    That they've so little of their art's
Knowledge, and don't understand
    What such a job of them demands
So that in these affairs so great
    Eternal life they take away
The earthly life I'll not lament
    Though it would be quite pertinent
So to my heart I've taken this
    In praise of God/ and to help us
To comfort also those poor souls
    Who with this will be saved twice-fold
And not so much death will occur
    As I have seen so oft before
Henceforth such carelessness shall be
    Avoided in human delivery
It'd come to the women quite easily
    How one can help a little baby
Midwives'll find their art here written
    What they should do with little children
I've given them what they must know
    Which they have in this small quarto
In it they'll find a good report
    Of what happens in human birth
If it be natural or no
    Dangerous/ bad/ or good/ also
What instruments they need to have
    So that the baby can be saved
And since no midwife that I've asked
    Could tell me anything of her task
I'm left to my medical education
    Which takes such things in consideration
I've put it down quite pleasantly
    In honor of feminine courtesy
    This must be understood verily
So women do not feel ashamed
    If they read all that it contains

And henceforth behave properly
    Before/ in/ and after delivery
For this book tells them thoroughly
    How they should act properly
    So that perhaps they won't miscarry
Much other help they'll also find
    Against miscarriage in womankind
And how to take great pains indeed
    The fruit inside their wombs to feed
Which the woman has conceived
    Who nat'rally her fruit conceived
Moreo'er one finds such evil women
    Who give to death a cause and reason
    That the fruit from life is driven
If God's a God on heaven's throne
    They'll reap from him what they have sown
    I'll leave these evil ones alone
This book is for the pious made
    Who will it close attention pay
And in their hearts seize upon this
    So that in their time of distress
They'll have to suffer much less woe
    And can much fear and pain forgo
For this book teaches excellently
    How one should practice skillfully
Nursing with care/ and also knowing
    The right way to act in all of these things.
¶I've given you ladies enough advice
    On how you'll come to recognize
Labor with ease and much less pain
    Just take to heart what I have penn'd
Though without pain you will not be
    Yet protected you'll better be
From miscarriage before the birth
    Your labor'll thus be easier
And so the name of this book is
    The pregnant woman's Garden of Roses
In which you dig and pluck the herbs
    Which have body, life/ and soul on earth
Such roses which your hands do take

Will come in time before God's face
Therefore you should take special care
 Have high regard and be aware
That the roses you select
 Are the ones that please God best
If after you leave this troubled existence
 You want to answer for your children
Then you will find here much of use
 And I will not ask more of you
Than to be honored in your thoughts
 As he who hath this garden wrought
For the ease and joy of the female sex
 I won't fight to earn more than that
And if such honor I am spurned
 I hope from God my praise to earn.

Prologue

After God the almighty/ in his high infinite wisdom/ created man from nothing/ out of merciful consideration so that he might have eternal joy and salvation/ He was inclined to him with such great love/ that out of the excess of his divine compassion/ He bestowed upon him so many blessings and gifts/ Graced him with so much reason and sense/ And so magnanimously shared the treasures of his infinite wisdom/ that man/ with the munificent help of the eternal wisdom/ has discovered the size width and breadth of the earth the seas and the air/ has measured the height and size of the heavens/ has observed the procession of the firmament/ the stars/ and the seven planets/ and has actually completely and certainly determined/ the path of the sun and also the moon. Thereupon these highly learned skillful scientists/ Galen/ Rhazes/ Avicenna/ Averroes and others whom it is not necessary to name/ were from the light of eternal wisdom/ so completely gifted and inspired and educated/ with such sharp reason and high understanding and with such clever sense/ that they/ through an infusion of divine grace/ and also with great deliberation/ industry and diligence/ were led to and have understood/ as much as is possible/ to keep a man healthy in his body/ And if he falls into sickness/ to cure him of it. Now when honorable modest women/ become pregnant/ their fruit might suffer much grief and suffering/ before/ during/ and after the delivery/ and various diseases and illnesses might befall them/ For example they are often burdened with children's afflictions/ with serious defects/ infirmities and calamities/ Because of which at times the poor suffering babies are wronged and cut off short/ so that they are robbed of holy baptism and eternal joy/ Therefore in honor and praise of the almighty God/ for the help and solace of poor suffering children/ and also for the love and service/ of honorable modest pregnant women this little handbook is published/ according to the above-mentioned highly learned and skilled scientists/ And it tells/ how one should remedy/ cure/ and avoid the illnesses/ diseases/ and misfortunes/ which befall and afflict/ pregnant-bearing women and their newborn children/ And this handbook is divided into twelve chapters.

Contents of the
Chapters of This Book

¶The tenth chapter tells/ how one should handle/ protect and tend the newborn baby/ and of its care.

¶The eleventh chapter tells/ how one should nurse the newborn child/ and how long/ also how the nurse/ and her milk should be.

¶The twelfth chapter tells/ of various troubles and illnesses of the newborn baby/ and how one may help it. And this chapter is divided into .xxxvi. parts.

The First Chapter
Tells How the
Baby Rests and Reposes in
the Womb / And How Many
Little Skins Surround and Wrap It

The baby rests in the womb thus. Its faced is bowed and bent quite close to its knees/ and it lays on its knees/ and has its nose between its knees/ and its eyes against its knees/ and is curled and bent like a round ball/ And its face/ and the front part of its body are turned toward the mother's back.

¶Furthermore in the womb the baby is hidden or wrapped up in three little skins. ¶The first skin surrounds and isolates the little baby and the other two skins/ On account of this the fetus is protected/ from harmful excess fluids of the woman's menstruation which remain/ after the woman has conceived/ and which are not fit or useful/ either for the nourishing or the growth of the baby/ Rather these same fluids of the woman's menstruation remain/ between the uterus and the first skin/ until the time of delivery/ Then at that same time they are cleaned away and driven out with the fetus and with the skin. And this first little skin is called in Latin Secundina/ and in German the "little bundle"*/ or afterbirth. And for the woman to be deliv-

---

*Buschelin. *The word Rösslin uses here means "little bush" or "little bundle"; he uses it variously to describe both the amniotic sac and the placenta. Soranus calls this the* "chorion, *because it contains* (kechorekenai) *the embryo and the things belonging to it"* (Soranus, p. 58). *For clarity's sake, throughout the rest of the text* buschelin *will be translated as "chorion."*

ered of the baby it is necessary/ for the skin to break open or be opened by the midwife/ as is written hereafter. ¶The second little skin called biles/ surrounds the baby/ from the navel down/ to the exit below/ and has many wrinkles and crooked twists or paths/ like a folded garment/ In this the urine/ sweat and other harsh things which come from the baby/ are collected/ held/ and enclosed/ until the time of delivery. Because of this the harshness of the urine and the sweat does not irritate/ or wound the baby or the first skin. For as long as the baby is in the womb it does not urinate through its genitals/ rather its urine flows through a little vein from the child's navel into the second skin/ of which we are now speaking. ¶The third skin/ lies closest to the child/ and completely surrounds it/ and protects the child from the harshness of its urine/ which flows out of its navel into the second skin through a small tube or vein. The third skin also protects the baby from the harshness of the first skin/ and the third skin/ as the great Albertus writes/ is called in Latin Armatura conceptus by midwives/ and in German a "baby's shield." Avicenna calls this skin amnios.

The Second Chapter
Tells of the
Time of Delivery and Which
Deliveries are Natural or Unnatural

When the time has finally passed/ before a woman should deliver/ which usually occurs in nine months so that the woman is near the fortieth week/ since she became pregnant/ then usually these signs appear. First the woman feels discomfort low in her body under the navel/ and in the back. Second, she feels pain in the joints near the genitals. Third, she has strong heat in her womb. Fourth/ the woman feels a tender swelling and moistness in her genitals as the uterus lifts. These are signs that the delivery is near. Then when the joints near the genitals swell up a great deal/ then the time for the birth has come. ¶It must further be known that there are two types of delivery. Natural and unnatural. The natural delivery is that/ which occurs at the right time with a correct position and a proper delivery. And the time of a natural delivery is usually in the .ix. month. At times although seldomly the delivery will occur when seven months have passed/ and the fetus may well remain alive after the birth. It can also happen that the child is born in the eighth month/ and the child rarely survives long after the delivery/ as Avicenna writes. Secondly, the natural birth should have the proper position. For Albertus Magnus writes that the baby should come out of the womb in the following manner. First the head/ then the neck and the shoulders/ so that the arms are extended down next to the sides of the legs/ and as the baby comes out of the womb its face is turned upward toward the heavens/ or toward its mother's navel. ¶As is shown here in the following figure.

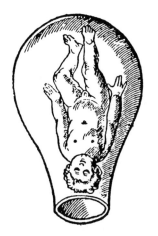

¶As Albertus Magnus writes and also as is written above/ the baby in the womb has its face and its breast against its mother's back before delivery and before it shoves itself/ And at the time of delivery the child pushes and throws itself over against its mother's back/ the head down by the opening/ and the feet up. Because of this in delivery the baby comes out with its face toward its mother's face.

¶Thirdly/ when it has come time for the delivery/ then in a natural birth the delivery of the child should be quick and easy/ without noticeable prolongation. This means that the unnatural birth is one which does not occur as has just been written. However Avicenna writes/ when a child comes out of the womb with the feet first/ and has its arms/ and its hands next to its sides extended down onto the thick part of its legs (as is drawn in this figure) that such a birth is unnatural/ yet it is the most similar of all to a natural birth/ because of the fact that it is not quite as dangerous as other unnatural births.

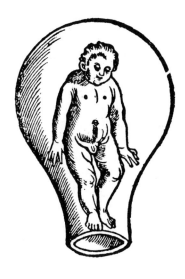

The Third Chapter
Tells Which
Deliveries Are Hard or
Easy / And How One Can and
Should Recognize Them

Here it must be known that frequently the delivery goes hard with much fear and danger/ and particularly great pain and suffering. And this happens in the first instance because the uterus is small/ and the woman has become pregnant before her twelfth year/ although that rarely occurs. ¶In the second instance the delivery is hard when the opening of the uterus is too narrow naturally/ or from afflictions and illnesses/ such as abscesses/ boils/ ulcers/ hemorrhages/ hemorrhoids. Because of these the uterus might not widen and open itself to a light and easy delivery of the baby without great pain. ¶In the third instance it is because of the fact that the woman's bladder/ entrails or intestines have abscesses/ ulcers/ boils/ or other injury and damage. Due to the pain they cause, the mother cannot easily be delivered of the fetus. ¶In the fourth instance it is due to the fact that her anus has boils/ chapping/ swelling of the veins which is called hemorrhoids/ or obstruction of hard compacted stools. And likewise if the woman is unable to push down/ this hinders the uterus in its action. ¶In the fifth instance it is because the woman is weak and of a sickly complexion/ or of a cold nature/ too young/ too old/ too fat/ too dry/ too thin/ has not had a child before/ and is fearful and intolerant of pain/ And also because she becomes restless and makes a quick movement from one place to another/ which brings her to and causes a troublesome hard delivery. ¶Sixth, it must be known that a boy is much easier to deliver than a girl. ¶In the seventh instance the delivery is hard and difficult/ if the baby is too big/ on account of which it cannot easily push through its mother's privates. Also when the child is too small and too light/ so that it turns and lowers itself down relatively less/ and is less easily pushed out.

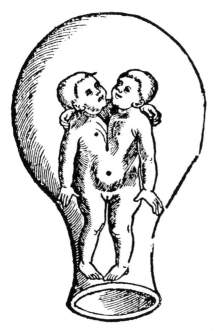

¶In the eighth instance/ it is because there is more than one baby/ or the baby has more limbs than is natural/ especially two heads as for example in this .xii. year in the county of Werdenberg/ a baby was born with two heads/ of which a figure is here drawn./ Or if the birth is too slippery/ so that it slips away and escapes from the pushing.

¶In the ninth instance/ the delivery will be hard if the child comes out in an unsuitable position/ like with both feet or knees/ or with one foot first. Also with the feet first and both hands raised up/ and this is the most hazardous delivery of all. Also if the baby's side appears first/ or the back or the bottom. Also if it is twins/ and both come with the feet first/ or one with the head first/ the other with the feet first/ And there may be many such unsuitable positions and unnatural deliveries/ as is described below in the fourth chapter. ¶In the tenth instance/ the delivery will be hard and difficult if the baby comes too soon especially in the third or fourth month/ at the time when the cords in the womb are holding strong and are tight/ as is written by Galen/ Also if the baby comes too late as in the tenth or eleventh month/ due to illness of the baby or its mother. ¶In the eleventh instance the delivery will be hazardous if the child is dead/ so that it cannot move itself to the opening/ Or if the child is sick and weak/ so that it cannot help itself to the opening. One should recognize as follows/ if it is sick in the womb/ Usually if the baby is sick in the womb/ then its mother has many illnesses/ too many bowel movements/ and much diarrhea/ for a long time without cease/ Or too much continuous bleeding/ after she has become pregnant. Also if the mother produces milk when you press her breast/ in the first month of her pregnancy. Likewise the child is sick/ when it does not stir and move very much at the time when it should be moving.

¶How one should recognize that the baby is dead in the womb, however/ and how one should remove it from the womb is written hereafter in the ninth chapter.

¶In the twelfth instance the delivery will be hazardous/ dangerous and hard/ if the chorion in which the baby lies/ is hard and tight/ and does not easily break/ Because of this the baby may not be able to get out/ Or if the chorion is too soft/ thin and delicate/ and quickly breaks/ before the baby has moved and shoved itself to the place of delivery/ So that the moisture and the water break and come before the proper time of delivery/ due to which the baby does not have moistness or slipperiness for a proper issuance. ¶In the thirteenth instance/ the delivery is hard if the woman suffers intense cold/ and the air is very dry/ so that the woman's womb becomes quite narrow/ as happens when cold winds blow. In addition the delivery is hard if there is intense heat/ for it weakens and enfeebles the baby/ as well as the mother/ so that neither of the two can help themselves in the delivery due to their feebleness. ¶In the fourteenth instance/ the delivery is hard if the woman has a habit of eating/ consuming and taking food and drink/ which dry and dessicate/ confine and tighten/ Like medlars/ chestnuts/ rowans/ wild plums/ millet/ rice/ and thick harsh red wine. ¶In the fifteenth instance/ the delivery is hard if the woman is near the time of delivery and has bathed over half her body/ in an alum bath/ iron bath/ salt bath/ in a cold bath or in a water bath/ in which things which press/ push and tighten have been boiled/ Like acorns/ oak bark/ acorn shells/ gall nuts/ pomegranate rinds/ dragonwort/ cinquefoil/ tormentil/ roses/ medlars/ wild pears/ crab apples/ flint/ and the like. ¶In the seventeenth instance/ as the woman approaches delivery/ the woman should not smell good-smelling things for the uterus will draw up toward the aroma/ and hinder the delivery. ¶In the eighteenth instance the birth is dangerous/ when the woman has great pains/ which do not go forward and down to the genitals/ but rather stay up in the body/ or go behind to the back. In addition labor is difficult and hard/ if it has been difficult and painful for the woman before/ as though it were her habit. ¶And the signs of a light easy delivery/ are contrary to the ones written above/ Like if the woman is wont to deliver lightly and easily/ and feels little pain at the time of delivery/ or a great pain which goes forward and down to the genitals. ¶Furthermore even if the delivery is hard/ there are still several good signs/ which give assurance of an auspicious delivery/ such as restlessness and movement of the child in the womb/ and when the labor pains move down out toward the genitals/ and the woman has a good strong robust breath/ with good strength in her body/ so that she can push down and labor well in the delivery. But the bad signs in a hard delivery are/ when the woman sweats a cold sweat/ and her pulse weakens rapidly/ and she becomes feeble and faints/ these are signs of a quick death.

The Fourth Chapter
Tells How a Woman
Should Behave During / Before /
and After the Delivery and
How One Should Come to
Her Aid in a Difficult Delivery

If one wishes to help with a difficult dangerous hard delivery/ which occurs with great sorrow/ anxiety/ and distress/ as has been reported above in eighteen passages in succession/ Then one must take note of what is written below. ¶The pregnant woman should follow two regimens. The first one month before the delivery. The second should be followed by the woman at the time of delivery. For the first she should avoid all things which hinder delivery/ if it is possible to do away with such things. If however they cannot be prevented or laid aside/ for example if the woman has such things naturally/ then as much as possible should skillfully be done/ in order to make the delivery easy. ¶Thus if the uterus/ or the woman's genitals are afflicted with boils/ ulcers/ warts/ venereal boils/ and the like/ on account of which the woman's genitals cannot widen and stretch due to pain/ then one should take counsel from a surgeon well before the delivery. Similarly if there is a problem of the bladder/ such as stones/ boils/ painful burning urination/ then one should take counsel beforehand and try to remedy the affliction. Also if the woman's anus is afflicted with warts/ hemorrhoids/ swelling/ abscesses/ ulcers/ and the like/ then one should take counsel before the delivery to remedy these. ¶Further if the woman has hard and compacted stools/ which make her bowel movements burn her/ then for one month before the delivery

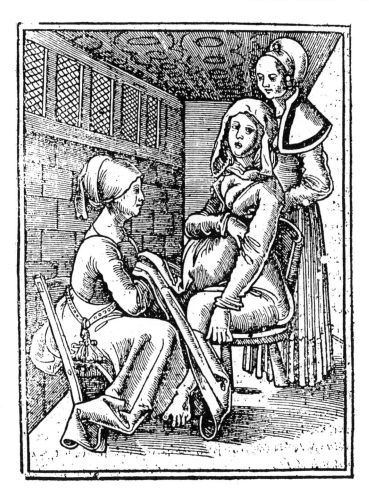

she should eat and drink things which soften and loosen/ Like baked apples with sugar eaten early/ with a glass of wine/ or with sweet apple juice. She might also want to eat figs mornings and evenings. And she should avoid those things that constipate/ like baked goods/ roasts/ rice/ hard boiled eggs/ millet/ and similar things. If necessary/ she can take a mild enema of chicken broth or meat broth without damage. She may also take a mild medicine to soften and loosen her stools. She can also use a suppository made of soap and fat/ or egg yolks. ¶Furthermore if the pregnant woman is feeble and weak as the delivery nears/ then one should begin to strengthen her beforehand with food and drink and with good electuaries. And after such things the woman should prepare herself and make herself fit and proper for the delivery with all the things that open/ widen/ soften and loosen/ and ease the openings of her genitals/ so that the genitals separate and let themselves be stretched and widened. And in particular women who have small and narrow genitals should do this. But in old women the genitals and uterus are drier and harder/ tighter and less able to be stretched apart than in young women. On account of this they should use things which are warm and moist and soften and smooth/ which are taken orally or introduced into the genitals/ or rubbed or salved externally/ Such as fatty meat broths/ particularly from young fat hens or capons. In addition she should use chicken fat/ duck fat/ goose fat/ oils which soften/ the slime which is made from quince seeds/ from dates/ from linseeds/ from althea/ or from fenugreek on her genitals. Also as the delivery nears the pregnant woman should drink good aged wine mixed with water. She should also have a regimen of food and drink. A regimen that moistens and does not produce too much fat/ and she should avoid that which dries/ constipates/ presses/ constrains/ tightens or narrows/ for one month before delivery. But if the woman gets very close to the time of delivery/ such that she has twelve or fourteen days until delivery/ and feels some heaviness and pain/ Then she should sit up to her navel in a water bath several times each day/ but not for too long (so that she does not become weak) And there should be things in this water bath that soften and smooth/ like mallows/ althea/ camomile blossoms/ dog's mercury/ maidenhair/ linseeds/ fenugreek seeds/ and the like. And if she cannot stand the bath due to weakness/ then she should still take a sponge or wool towel and wash her legs/ and her genitals/ private parts and hips with warm water in which the above-mentioned things have been steeped, and during this time she should not take a steam bath or go much in the public baths/ for she will become weak and feeble from these. And after the above-mentioned bath and washing the woman should take the oils mentioned before or a good fat marrow and smear/ rub/ and salve her back/ her body below the navel and at the sides/ and her legs right near the genitals. ¶Furthermore the woman should also put the above-mentioned fats/ oils/ and slime into her genitals in a sponge or cotton/ or in a little suppository sack by lying on her back/ her head low/ her rear end high/ so that the oils can get into her genitals. And in particular the woman should use these fats and oils in a sponge as is described above/ if the uterus is dry and dessicated/ or if the woman has a lean body. Furthermore she should make a good steam underneath of musk/ ambergris/ and gallia muscata*/ when you lay these on the coals it smells good/ and the uterus opens and goes down toward the good aroma. As the delivery approaches the woman should also eat small amounts of good foods/ which nourish and strengthen her well/ and she should drink good wine/ and should exercise with appropriate work/ and movement/ walking and standing more than she did before/ For such things will stimulate the birth.

The second regimen, which the woman should use at the hour of delivery/ when she experiences heaviness/ pain/ and various fluids which begin to appear and flow to the genitals/ has two parts. The first is/ to provide for an easy descent and delivery of the baby. The second is to alleviate the distresses, woes and pains of childbirth/ for this she should sit and then stand/ go up and down the stairs/ and yell out loud. Moreover the woman should push and force her breath out and also hold it in/ so that she presses and pushes her intestines down. ¶Furthermore the woman should also drink one of the medications listed below when she begins to push the baby out. After this when she feels the uterus open and the water flow copiously from the womb/ then she should lie down on her back/ but she should not lie down completely and yet she also should not quite be standing/ but rather it should be somewhere in the middle between lying and standing/ and the head should be lying more

French musk.

behind her than in front of her. And in high German lands/ and also in Italian lands the midwives have special chairs for a woman's labor/ and these are not high/ but carved out and hollow on the inside/ As depicted here. ¶And these should be made so that the woman can

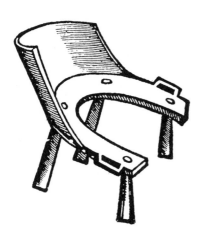

lean back on her back. ¶One should also pad the back of the chair with towels/ And when the time comes/ the midwife should lift up the towels well/ and turn the woman onto her right side/ and onto her left side, and the midwife should sit in front of her paying close attention to the movement of the baby in the womb/ and the midwife should observe the mother's organs and attend to them with hands/ smeared with white-lily oil or almond oil/ or the like/ and with the same hands the midwife should also gently take hold of the mother/ as she should rightly know. The midwife should also teach and counsel and advise the mother/ strengthen her with food and drink/ and with good, kind words urge the woman to labor/ and have her pull her breath in/ In addition to this the midwife should press gently on her stomach above the navel and the hips. The midwife should also promise the mother the happy delivery/ of a baby boy. And if the mother is fat/ then she should not sit/ rather she should lie on her belly/ and lay her forehead on the ground and pull her knees to her belly/ so that the womb is pushed and pressed. After that she should smear white-lily oil inside the genitals/ and if it is necessary then the midwife should take hold of her with her hands/ and widen the woman's privates/ and after this/ the woman will deliver quickly. Furthermore the midwife should begin no work with a delivering woman/ unless the baby appears and can be taken hold of/ or if she can see it/ for otherwise her work is in vain/ and the woman is sickened by it/ and overworks herself/ so that when she should labor she has become weak and sick. Now when the woman is in labor and the first skin in which the baby lies appears/ which is called the chorion/ or the after-birth/ then the delivery is nigh/ And if the skin won't break on its own because of its strength/ then the midwife should break it with her fingernail/ or she should grasp the chorion between her fingers/ and cut it open with a knife or a little scissors/ in such a way that she does not scratch or wound the baby. And after this the water will break out and the baby will follow. And if the midwife has cut open the chorion too early/ so that the water has all run out/ and the mother's genitals have dried up/ and the baby has not fully moved toward the opening/ and wants to prolong its delivery/ Then one should pour white-lily oil/ melted lard/ and fats in the proper warmth/ into the woman's genitals to make them smooth and slippery/ In particular egg whites/ with their yolks/ make a good medicine to pour into a woman's genitals in this emergency. And one should make her sneeze/ as this will bring on the delivery. ¶Furthermore if the baby is big/ and particularly the head/ then the midwife should gently widen the woman's genitals and the opening of the womb/ with her hands/ smeared with oil and fats that lubricate/ as written above. Similarly if the baby is a little daughter/ or twins/ then one should do with the oil/ as is written above.

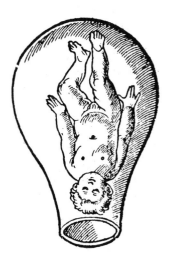

¶This is all written of a natural birth/ which is when the baby appears with its head first/ and the other limbs follow directly/ as is summarized above in the third chapter/ and indicated in this figure. ¶When however the baby appears and comes with an unnatural

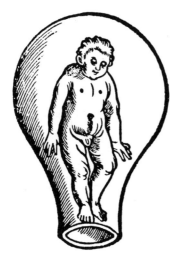

delivery/ with both feet first/ and with hands and arms extended down next to the legs as indicated in this figure/ then the midwife should properly guide/ adjust and turn the arms and hands of the baby/ with salves and other things that lubricate. Thus the hands and arms of the baby remain extended/ down next to the baby's sides on the thick part of its legs. And after this she should help it from its place. But wherever it is possible/ it is best if the midwife gently and tenderly guides the baby's feet up/ so that inside the womb the soles of the baby's little feet/ are shoved against the mother's navel/ and its little head is tilted and turned against its mother's back/ down toward the opening.

¶And when the baby appears with both feet first/ and does not have its hands next to itself/ extended down/ as described above/ but rather above its head/ Then the midwife should devote all her efforts to turn and bring the baby's hands down/ And where it is possible the midwife should turn the baby around/ in the same way as stated above/ and help it bring its head to the opening. But where this is not possible/ she should take it by the feet/ and guide the arms and hands down next to the sides/ and help it thus

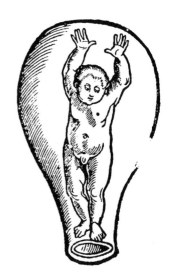

from its place/ And if these two ways are not suitable/ because of hindrances/ then the midwife should bind both feet of the baby together with a band of linen/ and then help the baby to the opening by pulling gently/ and this is the most dangerous delivery of all.

¶And when the baby comes out with only one foot first/ Then one should lay the mother on her back/ with her legs up/ her head down and her rear end lifted up high. And the midwife should gently shove the baby's foot back behind it with her hand/ And the mother should move herself around and roll a number of times/

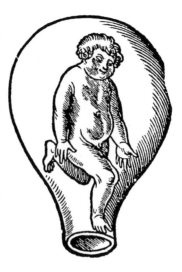

until the infant has turned its head down/ toward the opening/ After that the mother should sit up again on her chair and the midwife should help her as described above.

¶And if the baby will not turn in the womb so that the head comes down/ then the midwife should bring the other foot toward the opening also/ and help the baby come out/ but at all times with the arms and hands extended down next to its sides/ as described above.

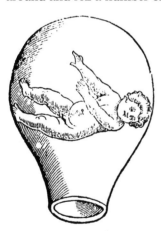

¶And when the baby comes to delivery with one side/ then the midwife should arrange/ adjust/ and direct the infant upside

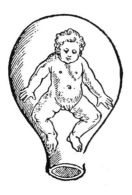

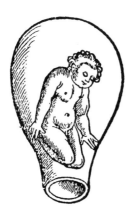

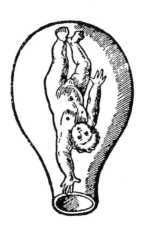

down/ the way it rested in the womb before/ and then help it to a proper issuance.

¶But if the baby comes out with its feet separated/ Then the midwife should put the feet together/ and then lead it out/ as is stated above. And at all times she should take great pains that the baby's hands are extended down next to its sides/ as has been written repeatedly here.

¶And if the baby presents itself by the knees/ or comes to delivery with one knee/ Then the midwife should lift the baby up and take hold of the feet/ and help the baby out as described above.

¶Furthermore if the baby presents a hand/ Then the midwife should not receive the baby/ rather she should put in her hand, take hold of the baby's shoulder, lift it back and extend the hand up next to the baby's side/ take hold of the head/ and help it out. But if such directing and arranging of the hand is unsuccessful/ Then it is necessary to lay the woman on her back/ with her head low and her behind high/ so that the infant falls down backward/ then sit her up again/ and help deliver the baby.

¶But if the baby appears with both hands/ then the midwife should take hold of both shoulders with her hands/ and lift the child back again/ And as is written above/ extend the baby's hands up next to its sides/ and then take hold of the head/ and help it out.

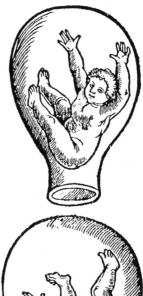

¶Furthermore if the baby presents its behind/ Then the midwife should put in her hand and lift the infant up/ and lead it out by the feet.

However where possible if she can shove the baby/ so it comes with its head down/ this would be much better than the first delivery.

Furthermore if the baby appears with a bowed/ inclined/ or crooked head/ The midwife should arrange the head properly and gently lift up the shoulders/ and bring the baby out.

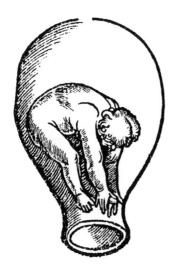

¶And if the baby comes with one or both feet/ and the head first/ Then the midwife should take hold of the head/ and direct the feet upward/ and thus help the infant to delivery.

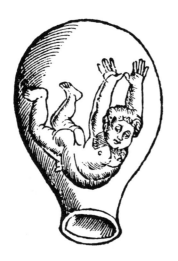

¶Furthermore if the baby lies akimbo or on its face/ then the midwife should gently insert her finger/ and turn the baby into the mother's side/ Or if she can insert a hand she should order and arrange the baby thus/ she should take hold of whatever part of the body is closest to the opening/ and lead it out/ but above all she should seek the head/ hold it and bring it out first.

¶Furthermore if the baby is more than one/ as in twins and both present their heads at the same time/ Then the midwife should bring them out one after the other/ in particular receive the first/ as stated above/ and do not forsake the second.

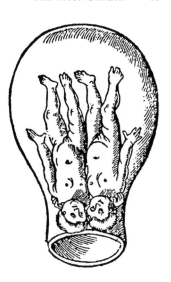

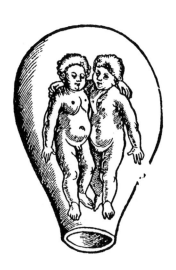

¶But if the twins come with the feet first/ then again she should take great pains/ to bring one out after the other/ just as is written above.

¶If however one of the twins comes with the head first and the other with the feet first/ Then the midwife should take care/ to help the nearest one first/ and not leave the other behind/ And this should be done/ without crossing the two.

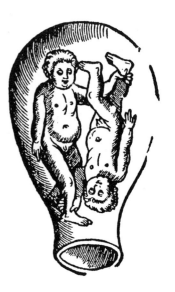

¶And if it is possible for the infant to turn itself around in the womb/ so that it comes with the head first/ this would be very good.

¶Thus the midwife should constantly sprinkle the woman's genitals with warm oils/ or with the slime from fenugreek seeds/ linseeds or mallow so that the baby may most easily be brought out/ and the woman might deliver with the least pain/ as also has been written above.

¶And if the mother has an abscess/ boil or ulcer in her genitals or womb/ and hasn't remedied them in time because of her proximity to delivery. Then into her genitals and womb you should pour oil/ fat/ and other things that will make them smooth and slippery/ in order to soothe the suffering and pain/ as is written above.

¶And this woman should lie on her stomach/ as was written earlier of a fat woman in delivery.

The Fifth Chapter Tells Which Particular Things and Medicines Aid the Delivery /
and Make It Light and Easy

The following things make a light and easy delivery. The woman who is delivering should sit down/ or lie on her back/ as is stated above/ each woman according to her custom. And if it is winter or otherwise cold/ then one should make the room or chamber warm. If it is summer or otherwise hot/ then one should air out the room and make it drafty/ so that the woman does not become too hot or faint. Furthermore one should also make the woman sneeze as stated above with hellebore/ or with powdered pepper or any other powder which causes sneezing/ And one should set her on a bench or chair as described above in the fourth chapter/ And the woman should push out her breath/ press/ lift/ and push down. Moreover one should press the woman's sides/ and push down. And the midwife should work diligently/ without stopping/ rather she should constantly apply oil and fat to the genitals and womb of the woman/ to make them slippery/ For this/ one should take duck fat or white-lily oil/ add to that two barley-corns weight of saffron/ and one barley-corn's weight of musk/ mix them all together well/ and salve the woman with it. And if this does not help then one should come to the woman's aid/ with smoke to the genitals/ of myrrh and galbanum and castoreum/ you should put all of these together with cow bile/ Take a dram's weight/ of these things you have put together/ and lay it on a small ember/ and let the smoke go up under the woman. Also another/ one should take

yellow sulfur/ myrrh/ madder which is used for making red
tints/ galbanum/ opopanax*/ mixed together with cow bile/ and
the woman should have her genitals fumigated with this smoke/
to aid delivery. Moreover if one fumigates her genitals with
dove dung/ it will also be quite good for her. Also fumigate her
genitals with opopanax/ and with hawk dung. ¶Also another/
One should moisten wool in rue juice/ and shove the wet wool
into the woman's genitals. Or you should place inside the wool
round birthwort/ or an herb called sowbread†/ or the seeds of
staphisagria/ called lousewort in English§/ and shove the wool
into the woman's genitals. Also one should wrap hellebore and
gum oppoponacum in wool and lay it in the woman's genitals/
for this thing drives and pulls the child living or dead from the
mother. Also the woman should take a bit of bark called cassia
fistula/ well pulverized/ and blend it into a brew of chickpeas or
wine/ and drink it/ this will make her deliver quickly. Also the
woman should take a gum called asafetida in Latin/ devil's dung
in English/ the size of a chickpea/ and add to it castoreum in the
size of a hazelnut/ or a dram's weight/ She should stir these two
in chickpea broth/ or in wine mixed with water/ and drink it.
Also it is good to drink cinnamon in wine or chickpea broth.
Also another/ Take water in which fenugreek seeds/ chickpeas/
and well-pounded maidenhair fern have been steeped/ stir into
this water syrup of roses with a little blue-lily oil/ and give it to
the woman to drink. Also take an herb called stone fern/ and
pound it well/ mix it with syrup of roses and a bit of oil and give
it to her to drink. Also take asafetida/ and a bark called cassia
fistula/ and give it to the woman to drink in wine. You should
also have the woman bathe in water in which you have steeped
althea. ¶In addition the following pill aids/ eases/ and lightens
the delivery/ Take a half lot each of cinnamon sticks and savin/
and one and one-half drams of the bark called cassia lignea**/
one dram each of myrrh/ birthwort/ costi amari*/ a shy half

*Oppoponacum: *juice of the panax (the herb ginseng).*
†*Cyclamen.*
§*Rösslin's text reads "in German," of course.*
**Senna.*

dram of storacis liquide†/ and one-fifth of a dram of a juice called opium/ make little pills of these/ and give the woman one-
half lot§ in four lots of good high-quality wine. Also saffron and
siler montan** make an easy birth in all animals to which it is
given. And if you give the woman saffron/ you shouldn't give
her more than a dram/ otherwise it is too much. ¶Also another
pill. Take five drams of savin, one and one-half drams of rue,
one-half lot of juniper berries, one-half lot each of asafetida, ammoniac, and madder used for coloring. Make a pill of these and
give the woman one-half lot to drink in water in which savin and
pennyroyal have been steeped, or with chickpeas and rue juice.
¶Another pill/ Take one-half lot of savin/ one-half dram each of
the gum called asafetida/ gum ammoniac and madder/ and
make a pill out of these with wine and give the woman one-half
lot to drink in wine. ¶Also another pill. Take equal amounts,
as much as you want, of birthwort/ called Aristolochia longa in
Latin/ pepper and myrrh/ make a pill with wine/ and give the
woman one-half lot with two lots of water in which lupines have
been steeped/ This is such a strong pill that it will make the
delivery light and easy/ and drive out whatever is in the womb/
be it living or dead. ¶Another pill just as strong as the last. Take
a gum called Bdellium/ which is white/ myrrh and savin/ make
pills the size of chickpeas out of these with cassia fistula and
honey/ give the woman five of these at once/ and this will lighten
and aid the delivery. ¶Also another medicine which has no
equal/ take a dram each of myrrh/ castoreum and storax/ make
pills out of this with honey and give the woman one-half lot at
a time in a drink of wine/ this is a powerful medicine.

¶Also a good plaster which aids delivery. Take colocynths/
simmer them in water and take the water and the juice of rue
and a little myrrh and a little barley flour/ make a plaster out
of these and lay it on the woman under the naval down to the

---

*Costus.
†Storax resin.
§A lot is an apothecary weight equal to one-half ounce. There are four drams in a lot.
**Bastard lovage.

genitals/ it helps well. And although there are still many more things that aid the delivery/ and make it easy and light/ the most valuable of these are described above/ and the others have been omitted for brevity's sake.

The Sixth Chapter Tells How
One Brings Out the Chorion Which Is the Afterbirth from a Woman When It Won't Come Out by Itself During Delivery

Here it must be known that at times the chorion or afterbirth comes out with the baby/ at other times it stays behind/ because the baby is born under such difficult circumstances/ that the mother is sick and weak after the delivery and not strong enough to push the chorion out with vigor. Or because the chorion is tightly fastened and fixed inside the womb. Or because of the fact that after the water has flowed during delivery/ the chorion is left dry in the womb without the moisture which should give it a slippery path to the exit. Or because the opening of the womb is narrowed/ tight/ and swollen due to pain. ¶If then the chorion has stayed behind for whatever reason/ Then the midwife should take serious and diligent action to bring the chorion out from its place/ for if this does not happen/ then the woman may fall into great sickness/ in particular into a suffocation from the womb/ which is called suffocatio matricis in Latin. And this is because/ when the chorion remains behind/ it rots easily by nature/ and from it evil vapors go up to the mouth of the woman's stomach/ to the heart/ into the head/ and to the skin above which the lungs and heart lie/ which is called dyafragma in Latin. Because of this the woman becomes short of breath and tight-chested/ and faints and lies as if she were dead/ so that one often finds no pulse/ and at times she chokes and dies. Therefore in order to prevent such great illness/ the midwife should assist in bringing the chorion from its place. ¶If the chorion remains behind due to weakness in the mother/ then one should strengthen her with food and drink and other invigorating things/ such as good broth from egg yolks/ wine/ meat/ chicken/ birds/ partridges/ hazelhens/ young turtledoves/ capons &c. And thus the woman should be strengthened as is reported above on the difficult delivery which is due to the woman's weakness. ¶Furthermore if the chorion stays behind due to a narrow closing and swelling of the womb/ Then one should use things that make it smooth and slippery and open the womb, like the oils, fats, &c. which are described above on the difficult delivery &c. Furthermore white-lily oil, marjoram oil, oil from the daffodil called narcissus in Latin, and blue-lily oil/ all open the womb. ¶Also juniper berries/ and a gum called galbanum pulverized and steeped in warm wine and drunk is good for a narrow womb. Southernwood or lad's love drunk warmed in wine is also good. In addition pennyroyal soaked in wine and drunk widens the womb and drives the chorion to a proper issuance. Also good for widening the womb/ are the things that make it mild and soft/ like chicken fat, goose fat, duck fat/ and lily oil poured in and rubbed inside and out-side. It is also good for the woman to warm herself or make a vapor/ or a steam with mallows/ althea/ bearsfoot/ and bran/ or bathe in this/ or make a little sack out of it and lay it in the genitals. ¶Furthermore if the chorion is too firmly attached or fixed to the womb/ so that the bonds won't let loose/ Then the woman should fumigate herself from below with sulfur/ ivy leaves/ and watercress. It is also good for her to warm herself with watercress and figs. Furthermore all things that smell good/ like ambergris/ musk/ thimiama gallia muscata/ and a confection called confectio nere/ should be laid on coals by the woman/ and she should fumigate herself from below to the genitals/ and cover herself well/ so that the good smell does not come up to her nose/ Rather the woman should smell things that smell evil and stink/ And she should make a vapor for her nose from things which smell evil and stink/ such as asafetida/ cas-toreum oil/ burned human hair/ and burned peacock's feathers

&c. Also the woman should fumigate up into her genitals with smoke made from asses' hooves/ and no matter how evil the smoke smells/ it has by nature the property/ of pulling out the dead baby/ and also the chorion. ¶Furthermore the woman should hold her breath/ and push down/ one should also make her sneeze with hellebore or with ground pepper while holding the mouth and nose shut/ And push down on her sides with the hands/ so that the chorion is led forth toward the opening. Also a salve called ungentum basilicon*/ of which Mesue writes in the .xi. section/ should be poured into the womb/ for this salve softens/ and brings forth the chorion/ and pulls it down to the opening/ and when the chorion has come out/ then one should pour rose oil in the womb. It is also good to take good rose water with powdered althea/ and drink it for such a thing makes the chorion slip softly out. ¶Furthermore when some of the chorion appears/ Then the midwife should softly pull so that it does not break off/ and if it is in danger of breaking/ then the midwife should bind as much as she has hold of/ on the top of the woman's leg/ not too tight or too loose/ but to the proper degree so that it does not break/ and so that on the other hand it does not pull back in/ And one should make the woman sneeze/ as is written above. And if the chorion only lengthens/ and does not go out/ then you should not stretch it fully or pull it/ rather bind it on top of both legs or some other place/ so that it does not rise up/ And if it is tightly fixed in the womb then the midwife should delicately peel it out without causing great pain in the woman/ and she should not pull down hard so that the womb does not come out after it/ Rather she should pull cautiously or pull to the side from one side to the other/ here a little and there a little until it is well freed/ After that she should pull until it is completely peeled from the womb to which it is fixed and help it out. Furthermore if the chorion delays too long in the womb, so that the woman gets very sick from it, or a headache, fainting &c. Then one should give her things that strengthen the head and the heart/ good for this are electuaries/

*A salve made from walnuts.

which contain musks/ like diamuscum/ dyambra/ confectio de gemmis/ dyamargariton and others.* For this one should resort to the doctors. Also things that strengthen the stomach/ like dyagalanga/ dyacinamomum/ and others which one finds in the apothecaries/ And it is good to take such electuaries and confections with wine. ¶Also another thing with which one drives out the chorion. Take equal amounts of rue/ horehound/ which is called marrubium/ prassium in Latin/ southernwood or lad's love/ mugwort or sailor's tobacco/ and take enough lily oil so that the herbs all become well moistened/ and put it all in a glass pot and cover it tightly with a lid which has a little hole on top/ and make a hollow tube to fit in the little hole/ and let the pot with the things boil/ and when it comes to a good boil then take the pot from the fire/ and set it on warm embers under a bench upon which the woman sits/ and take one end of the tube/ and stick it in the little hole on top of the lid so that the steam does not go out/ and the woman should put the other end of the tube in her genitals/ and she should cover herself with cloth and wool so that no steam gets out, and she should sit like this for two hours until the chorion removes itself. And if such steaming still does not help then the woman should lay a plaster/ on her body between the genitals and navel/ which has the power to drive out a dead infant/ and which will be described below. And if the chorion still does not come out after all of the above-described methods/ then one should not expend any more care or work with it. For in a few days it will flow out and go away/ like a spongy water. But if the chorion stays a long time/ and then flows out/ then its odor will bring alarm/ headaches/ weakness of the stomach/ and heartsickness to the woman/ as described above.

---

*These are all compositions found at the apothecary. "Dyagalanga," for example, was a mixture of "Galanga, wood aloes. . . . Cloves, Mace, seeds of Lovage . . . Ginger, long and white Pepper, Cinnamon, Calamus Aromaticus . . . Calaminth, and Mints dried, Cardamoms the greater, Indian Spicknard, the seeds of Smallage, Annis, Fennel, [and] Carraway" (Nicholas Culpepper, Pharmacopoeia Londinensis, by Peter Cole, 1659, p. 233).

The Seventh Chapter
Tells of Various
Conditions Which Come and Befall a
Woman During and After the Delivery,
and How One Should Remedy Them

Of the conditions and illnesses which follow the delivery/ it must be noted that usually after the delivery the woman has such conditions/ as fever which is unnaturally high heat/ puffing or swelling in the body/ pain in the body/ and movement of the womb or displacement of the womb. And the usual cause of the condition is incomplete cleansing of the blood after the delivery/ and weakness of the woman's vigor/ due to a great loss of blood after the delivery. Also due to injury/ tearing/ and rupture of the womb/ or various veins in the womb/ or due to pain from protrusion of the anus. If a full flow of blood does not come out of the woman after the delivery as it should/ Then one should help her with things that bring on the flux/ as many honorable women well know/ among these are/ foot baths/ warming/ sulfur/ fumigation to the genitals/ laying plaster on the body/ steeping herbs and binding them on/ salving and the like/ according to the circumstances. One should take pains to completely cleanse the woman with warm things that drive out the urine. For all things which drive out the urine bring the woman her natural time of the month/ and also cleanse her blood flow after delivery/ since these are what make the blood flow out/ and because of these the veins widen so that the blood might flow/ and drive the matter down and out/ These things are mugwort or sailor's tobacco, hazelwort, savin, pennyroyal, parsley, chervil, anise, fennel, juniper, rue, laurel leaves, germander/ valerian/ cinnamon sticks/ spikenard/ and many other things/ But one should use these things under the advice of a wise learned doctor/ so that the heat does not become too great. Also if the woman wants to increase her flow of blood/ she should sneeze a lot/ holding the mouth and the nose closed as she sneezes and hold her breath and push down. She should also place a cup or cupping glass inside both legs above the knees near the genitals and draw the blood. Or she should make a vapor with salted fish eyes or from horses' hooves or asses' hooves/ and let the vapor go up to her genitals. And if this does not help/ then if the woman is strong enough/ she should let blood from the woman's vein called saphena in Latin/ under the ankle bone inside the foot/ for this very letting brings on the woman's menstruation. ¶And if the woman gets a fever after delivery/ that is unnaturally high heat/ then it is good for her to let the woman's vein/ or the vein under the ankle bone as described above/ for fever usually befalls a woman after delivery due to a hindering of the menstruation which would be brought forth through such bloodletting. Also in fever she should drink barley tea made from steeped husked or crushed barley. Or water in which chickpeas and barley have been steeped together. She should also drink whey/ or a water in which tamarisc/ which is a black sour fruit similar to plums/ has been steeped. She should also take good chicken broth and eat sweet pomegranate/ for such things bring on a woman's menstruation/ cool the unnatural high heat and soften her body if it was stopped up before. ¶When however it befalls a woman after delivery that her body becomes puffed and swollen/ then she should drink chickpea water with powdered roman caraway. Or a good wine with an electuary called dyamarte/ or one called alkakengi of which Avicenna writes in the fifth book/ as the doctors well know. Or she should use a gum called serapinum/ and dittany or borage and mastic. Also good are enemas made from things that consume and drive away the gas and wind or a little suppository that one puts in the genitals/ called pessarium in Latin/ made from round birthwort and from squinante*/ from

*Camel's hay.

storax liquida/ from leopard's bane/ and from zedoary &c. Furthermore if after delivery the woman gets sickness and pain in her body/ her womb and her genitals/ Then she should warm herself or bathe with things that lessen the pain/ like mallows, althea, fenugreek, roman caraway, camomile blossoms, blind nettles which are called our lady's slippers/ and resemble the dead nettle with white-yellow colored blossoms, and an herb called water hemlock. Also good for pain is for a woman to rub and smear herself with oil from sesame or sweet almond oil.

¶Furthermore if she does not have great heat/ she should use treacle or a confection called triffera magna/ in wine in which red mugwort or an herb called camomile or matricaria in Latin has been steeped. ¶Also another thing which is good for pain in the genitals. Take pennyroyal/ an herb called policaria* in Latin/ and six bay leaves/ and let them all boil/ and have the woman warm and steam herself over it. ¶Also another thing to lessen the pain and discomfort of the genitals after delivery/ Take rue/ red mugwort/ and southernwood or lad's love/ pound them well with pennyroyal oil/ and put it all together/ and heat it in a pot/ and wrap it all in a cloth/ and lay it on the woman's genitals. ¶Also another thing for pain of the genitals after delivery. Take four handfuls each of camomile blossoms and linseeds/ pound the seeds and put it all together in a little sack/ simmer it in white wine and lay it warm on her body. ¶Also another/ give the woman two barley-corns' weight of musk in wine to drink. ¶Also another/ Take white onions and lay them in hot ashes/ then peel them and pound them well/ and add to them unrefined dairy butter without salt/ and make it into a plaster/ and lay it warm on her body. Also fumigate her underneath to the genitals with frankincense and storax. ¶And if the woman has great pain in her back after delivery/ Then one should take two handfuls each camomile blossoms/ and blind nettles/ and one handful each/ wormwood and southernwood/ three handfuls mugwort/ one lot each cinnamon bark/ powdered nutmeg/ steep these things in water through three or four

*Fleabane.

boilings/ and with the same water soaked into a bath sponge/ the woman should warm her back well/ or put all the things in a little sack/ and bind it warm onto her back. And if this is not of enough benefit/ Then take three lots each of spikenard and white-lily oil/ one dram of powdered nutmeg/ and mix these things together/ and rub it well into the back. Or take two lots each of dill oil/ camomile oil/ four lots of white-liy oil/ and one-half a lot of wax/ melt these things together over a fire/ and make a salve out of it/ and rub and smear the woman with this as above. ¶Furthermore if after delivery the woman's menstruation flows too much and too heavily so that she becomes quite weak and feeble/ Then it must be known that the excessive flow of the woman's menstruation comes from various causes. First from superfluous blood in the whole body. Second due to much mixing of the gall with the blood/ so that the blood becomes sharp and hot/ and because of this it widens and courses through the veins and then goes into the womb. Third because the blood is too watery and thin and thus courses quickly. Fourth/ because the veins are large/ so that the release of blood becomes increased. Fifth/ because the womb is so weak/ and the veins so loose and wide that they cannot hold the blood. Sixth because the entire body has such solid and compact hard flesh that the sweat holes are narrow and closed or stopped up/ so that not much sweat/ steam/ or vapors come from the body and consequently moisture and fluid collect inside the body which then increase the woman's menstruation and flow out with it. Seventh/ because some certain veins in the womb open/ which are called hemorrhoids. Eighth/ because inside the womb are tears/ abscesses/ or boils. Ninth/ because the woman has fallen/ or has been struck or hit or thrown behind on her bottom or forward on her genitals. In the tenth instance the woman's menstruation becomes heavy/ if the womb is torn or injured during a difficult delivery. ¶Thus since there are various causes for a woman's excessive bleeding/ it is very important that the woman in distress not have too much shame/ rather she should disclose and explain her concern to the doctor. From his questions and her answers this doctor may well be informed of the cause by which she has excessive flow/ according to which he can advise her properly. ¶Although there are many medicines which cure such bleeding/ such as electuaries/ confections/ trocisci*/ drinks/ powders/ suppositories/ fumigation/ warming/ baths/ plasters/ and lotions/ about which many honorable women are well informed/ Following for the help and comfort of the dear woman is a list of a few particular medicines against excessive flow of the woman's menstruation. ¶First if the woman's bleeding is too heavy/ then one should bind her arm very hard, as much as she can stand/ and not the foot or the leg/ and one should set a large cupping glass or a drinking glass under her breast/ but without pricking. And one should moisten cloths in vinegar and lay them on her body under the navel and above the genitals/ and also lay things in the genitals/ which stop blood/ like pomegranate flowers/ or the skin of pomegranates/ yellow amber/ terra sigilata†/ bolus armenus, a red earth§/ dragon's blood/ bloodstone/ called ematites in Latin**/ red roses/ frankincense/ and oak apples/ you should take all these things/ or as many as you might have/ of each an equal amount/ and powder them finely/ and make a plaster out of them with thick red wine/ and put the plaster in a little sack/ one finger long and a thumb thick/ and put a little fat on the sack and put the sack in the genitals. ¶Also another plaster which is good/ on the body and on the genitals take one lot each of bloodstone/ called ematites/ and bolus armenus/ one-half lot each of dragon's blood/ and a juice called licium††/ a dram each/ of yellow amber/ acorn shells/ cypress nuts/ and pomegranate flowers or the skins/ one and one-half dram/ of flint from the blacksmith/ equal amounts of turpentine/ and colofonia/ which is scammony/ enough to make a plaster/ with the above things well pounded and pulverized. ¶Also a salve for the same thing/ Take one-half pound each of an oil called oleum mirtinum*/ and rose oil/ two lots each

---

*Troches are little cakes which were found in the apothecary. See Culpepper, pp. 268–69.
†Lemnian earth.
§Armenian bole.
**Hematite.
††A medicinal powder made from the dried juice of certain plants (Rowland, p. 11ff).

of yellow amber/ scrapings from elephant bone/ scrapings from goat horn/ red coral/ terra sigillata/ and frankincense/ five lots of white wax/ make a salve out of all these which the woman can rub and smear on her body and also her genitals. ¶In addition a bath/ in which the woman should sit up to her navel. Take two handfuls each of wormwood/ lance-leaved and broad-leaved plantain/ and the sour knobs on the grapevine/ and the young shoots from the blackberry bush/ unripe plums/ unripe sloes/ unripe wild pears/ medlars/ three handfuls of red rose leaves/ four handfuls of oak bark/ two handfuls each nightshade/ and Fuller's teasel/ a good handful each of cinquefoil grass and root/ tormentil/ dragonwort/ a bowl full of acorn husks/ two handfuls each of oak apples and shelled acorns/ and bursa pastoris/ called shepherd's purse in English/ One should pound these things to a powder and the excess should be cut into small pieces and all should be boiled in rain water/ or in water in which .x. or .xii. flints have been extinguished three times/ And finally she should bathe in this water/ until the bath is tepid. And when she gets out of the bath/ if she has a great thirst she should take one-half lot of the electuary athanasia or micleta with plantain water/ or if she is not thirsty she should take it with thick red wine. Furthermore this electuary is also good/ take four lots of rose sugar/ one-half lot each of red coral/ burned elephant bone and bolus armenus/ three drams bloodstone/ You should pulverize these things finely and mix with sugar roset†/ and take one-half lot/ mornings and evenings with plantain water/ or with shepherd's purse water. Also another/ take bloodstone/ rub it on a whetstone and wash the stone with plantain juice until the juice becomes red/ give her two or three spoonfuls of the juice to drink early in the morning. Also good for this are little cakes from the apothecary/ called trocisci of yellow amber or trocisci of bolus armenus/ blend a dram of this or a little more/ with five spoonfuls of plantain water and give it to her to drink.

Myrtle oil.
†*A candy made of a distillation of rose juice, rose leaves, and sugar (Culpepper, p. 221).*

¶And whoever wishes to be further informed in these things/ should take counsel with the doctors. ¶Furthermore if after the delivery/ the woman gets ulcers/ abscesses/ boils or the like/ in the womb or the genitals/ then one should clean the boils/ and lessen the pain with the juice from dried nightshade berries/ and with broad-leaved plantain juice and with rose oil/ Temper these things well among one another/ and pour it on the woman's boils/ or lay it on with cotton. Also another/ Take the white of an egg/ and mother's milk and purslane juice and temper it all together/ and do as described above. Also another/ The woman should sit up to the navel in a bath/ in which pomegranate rinds/ red rose leaves/ acorn husks/ oak bark/ tormentil/ dragonwort and cinquefoil grass and root have been boiled. ¶Furthermore if the boil is cleaned and purified/ then one should rub it with a salve/ the white or the red salve which they make in the apothecary or with other salves which cool and heal. ¶And the way one helps a woman if she has boils/ as described here/ is also how one helps her if the womb or genitals are injured. ¶But if after the delivery/ the woman's rectum comes out then the midwife should warm her hand in good white wine/ and then with warm hands carefully push the rectum into its proper place. And if the rectum is swollen/ then she should melt unrefined butter in wine/ and moisten cotton in this and apply this to the rectum and warm it until it shrinks. Or one should shrink the swollen rectum with cotton soaked in warm milk. And when it is shrunk then one should push it in/ as described above/ and one should shove the rectum in with a round ball of wax/ melted with mastic or frankincense/ and wrap a bandage over it so that the wax may not move. And this should be done as often and every time the woman has a bowel movement/ until the rectum is well secured and no longer comes out. And if one does not want to use wax/ then you should take cotton and make it round/ and moisten it in mastic oil or nard oil and lay it very warm on the rectum/ and then bind it/ as described above. ¶Also another/ wash the rectum with water in which things that dry and absorb have been boiled/ such as oak apple/ cypress nuts/ pomegranate rinds/ yellow amber/ mastic/

frankincense/ and dragon's blood/ Then sprinkle pulverized burned hartshorn on the rectum and push it in/ as described above. ¶Furthermore if the woman's womb comes out after delivery/ Then you should warm the womb with warm water in which these things have been boiled/ Take two lots each cypress nuts/ red roses/ spikenard/ pomegranate rinds and also the flowers/ and acorn husks/ a handful each of unripe medlars/ unripe rowans and apples/ unripe plums/ and sloes/ pound the things which can be powdered well and cut up the herbs/ boil all the things in rain water if you have it or in mineral water and make a bath up to the navel/ or warm the uterus with a sponge or cotton soaked in the water. Then dry it with a soft white cloth and trickle on it this powder pounded fine/ and sieved through a silk cloth. Take frankincense/ yellow amber/ oak apple/ pomegranate rinds and flowers/ cypress nuts/ alum/ antimony, bolus armenus, and mastic/ sprinkle this powder on the uterus and then put it in and bind it with a warm cloth. If however the uterus has become hard and swollen then you should shrink it and make it warm with good white wine in which butter has been melted/ Then put it in as described above/ and put two cupping glasses against the body above and on each side of the genitals/ and lay the woman on her back with her rear end very high/ and use the above-described powder and binding as long as it takes until the uterus stays in the woman and no longer comes out. ¶Furthermore if the woman's navel comes out after delivery/ then take a fine pledget and wrap it with a fine soft cloth/ and take well-powdered frankincense/ and temper the powder with egg white/ so that it becomes like a fluid honey/ fill inside the navel with this same powder and egg white/ and rub it in/ and moisten the pledget in the same thing and shove and push it in the navel/ and bind the pledget and the navel together. ¶Finally sometimes it happens that during a hard/ difficult/ dangerous/ and delicate delivery/ the woman suffers great distress in that the genitals and anus tear and fall together/ and the uterus comes out. And that is because/ if the woman's genitals through which the baby should go/ are too narrow and delicate/ and the baby is big/ the genitals are pushed/ forced/

and pressed so hard that such breaks occur. Now first the pushed-out uterus is to be warmed/ washed/ heated/ shrunk/ and pushed in/ as is described above in the part before last. Then one should give the tear between the genitals and the anus four or five stitches/ as many as necessary/ with a strong silk thread. ¶Also if you want to help her in another way without stitches and without sewing the skin/ then. One should take two strong pieces of linen as long as the tear and two fingers wide/ which have no seams along the length but have a finished edge. Onto these two cloths one should smear a strong plaster that holds and sticks well/ and one should lay one on the right side near the tear/ lay the other on the other side along the length of the tear. So now the plaster is spread on well/ and it sticks and holds fast to the skin/ so that the skin or the flesh of the tear peeks out from under the cloth by the thickness of a rye straw or a bit more. Then one should sew the cloths together with a strong thread/ but do this so as not to touch the skin. As the surgeons should know/ this is how you bring the lips of the tear together. After this you should place fluid pitch on it. ¶Also another remedy for the above-described tear/ Take comfrey/ called con- solida major in Latin/ dry it well/ and pound it to a powder. Then take powdered roman caraway and pounded cinnamon sticks/ mix them all together/ and put this powder on the woman's tear and in her genitals.

The Eighth Chapter Tells
of Miscarriages of the Baby /
and Causes and Signs of Miscarriage.
Also of Problems After the Miscarriage /
and How One Should Avoid Them &c.

A miscarriage of a baby is nothing other than a delivery or birth of a premature baby. And this happens many ways. Sometimes it happens before the creation of the baby and before it receives its soul. Sometimes it happens after the soul has been imparted/ and before the baby stirs and moves/ that is before the time is half passed. Sometimes it happens after the halfway point in time before the baby moves and before a full completion of the time to delivery/ so that the baby is usually dead when it comes out of the mother's body too early/ although occasionally it is alive/ and this premature or unnaturally early delivery of a baby has many causes. For example it is due to the womb/ if the entrance to the womb/ which is called interius or matricis in Latin/ is too slippery/ too smooth/ and too soft due to bad fluids which flow there. Or because the womb is unsuitable/ loose/ and full of moisture inside/ so that it cannot keep hold of the male seed/ or the baby it has received. Or because the womb is burdened with some sickness/ such as boils/ ulcers/ abscesses/ and the like. Or because the veins and the cord of the womb to which the baby is attached/ and through which the baby receives its nourishment/ are stopped up with slimy fluids, or are broken by bad gases/ as a result of which the baby cannot have its nourishment/ and is driven to delivery/ after the second or third month. For as Hippocrates says/ Those women who have suitable bodies/ not too fat and not too thin/ and who become pregnant and miscarry in the second or third month/ without apparent cause/ in such women the cord which holds the baby in the uterus/ called cotilidones in Latin/ is full of evil slimy fluids/ so that it breaks/ and cannot hold the fetus because of its weight. Avicenna adds to this that women usually miscarry in the second and third month from gases and moisture of the veins that are in the uterus. In addition women sometimes also miscarry due to illnesses of the organs/ which push against or are near the womb/ for example if the rectum is burdened with ulcers/ boils/ and hemorrhoids. Or if the bladder has stones/ boils/ ulcers/ or burning &c. And if these are the cause/ then the intense/ hard/ excessive pushing which occurs with diseases of the rectum and bladder/ cause severe downward movements/ which makes the birth cord break and let go. ¶Miscarriages also come from an illness which is called tenasmon in Latin/ and this is an illness in which/ one has a constant desire to pass stools and pushes and forces/ and yet accomplishes little or nothing at all. Hippocrates says of this that/ Those women who are pregnant and afflicted with this illness/ usually miscarry their babies. ¶Moreover women also miscarry from severe heavy coughing/ as Hippocrates also writes. Women who are pregnant who are too gaunt and skinny/ usually miscarry before they gain weight. And the reason says Avicenna/ is that women who are pregnant and emaciated/ need the food that they eat/ to support and replenish or nourish their bodies. Because of this there is not enough food left over to nourish the baby in the mother's body. As a result the baby becomes weak in the womb/ and does not want to stay/ but rather is forced out. ¶Women also miscarry if they bleed too much or have had their monthly times too often. On this matter Hippocrates says if a woman is pregnant/ and bleeds/ then it is impossible for the fetus to be healthy. This should be understood/ if the woman's menstruation is heavy/ and the woman does not have a strong body/ especially if she is small and thin. Also if her monthly time comes to her after the third month/ for in the first and second month the woman may well bleed without damage to the fetus/ because the fetus is small and does not need much nourishment. ¶A woman also miscarries as Hippocrates says if she has her blood let/ that is to say/ if the woman is not rich in blood/ if however she has more blood than she and the baby need/ then she may let blood after the fourth month and before the seventh/ but she should not let blood without necessity and good reason. ¶A woman also miscarries if she uses harsh medicines to pass stools before the fourth and after the seventh month/ But if it is necessary for the woman to purge herself/ which should only occur for noteworthy reasons/ then it would be least dangerous and damaging to the fetus/ between the fourth and seventh months/ and it should be done gently with subtle and soft medicines/ as Hippocrates says. ¶It is also common for a woman to miscarry/ if she is struck by bad dysentery. For Hippocrates says/ if a woman is pregnant/ and has a great deal of diarrhea/ then there is a danger that she will miscarry/ this should be understood to mean a bad chronic diarrhea/ in a thin woman. Because the woman's blood decreases/ and she becomes sick/ so that the fetus is forced to come out/ due to lack of food. ¶Moreoever a woman miscarries if she vomits or becomes sick a great deal. For Avicenna says/ that vomiting and the distress of vomiting makes women thin/ consumes them/ and can break the birth cord/ because of the excessive movement of vomiting. ¶Also women who suffer from extreme hunger miscarry/ or those who are stricken by a serious dangerous illness. Hippocrates speaks of this thus/ It is deadly/ if a woman is pregnant and gets a bad disease/ like the pestilence/ growths on the breast/ a stroke/ falling sickness/ or a serious harsh fever. ¶Women also miscarry due to great gluttony/ which suffocates the baby in the womb/ and makes the baby's nourishment improper/ for gluttonous eating cannot be digested and does not make good blood/ from which the baby should be nourished. ¶Also the woman can miscarry because the baby is very weak and sick/ from things inside or out which can make it sick or kill it/ so that the womb becomes burdened/ and tries to push the baby out. ¶Moreover a woman can miscarry if the chorion or skin/ in which the baby is wrapped breaks too early/ because it is weak and cannot hold the baby.

Or if the womb's moisture flows/ and makes the uterus slippery and provokes and promotes the delivery of the baby. ¶A woman also miscarries from intense excessive coldness in the air which kills the baby/ as occurs in the country around the time of midnight/ or from intense heat/ which makes mother and baby weak/ this happens especially in hot countries around midday. Thus pregnant women should not bathe much/ nor stay long in a bath/ for three reasons. First, because she can get short of breath due to the bath. Second, because the bath makes the fetus's cord soft/ widens the birth canal and makes it smooth and slippery/ and because of this the delivery gives way. Third, because the baby becomes too hot in the mother's body/ so that it is driven out in order that it may have cool air. Consequently she should neither bathe much nor long/ if she is pregnant/ but only as much/ as is described above regarding difficult births/ and how women may ease them through bathing. At that time it was also said/ that the safest way would be/ for the woman who is approaching the time of delivery/ to wash her legs as stated above/ so that she would soothe the excessive heat of her body. ¶Women also miscarry/ if the season changes/ or turns contrary to the usual course of nature. For Hippocrates says/ that if there is a warm wet winter/ followed by a cold dry spring/ the women who should bear in spring easily miscarry/ due to minor causes. And if they do not miscarry/ then they deliver sickly children/ who die quickly/ or live weak unhealthy lives. And this is the reason/ in that winter the woman's body is warm and moist/ and opened up from the warmth or wetness of the winter/ as if she had been in a warm bath. Thus the cold of the following spring easily penetrates her body/ Now when the baby in the womb becomes accustomed to warmth in the warm winter/ and then the cold spring quickly follows then the cold penetrates the baby/ so that it dies in the womb or shortly after it has been born into this world. And if it lives/ then it will hardly be able to endure and survive such a great change and transformation from warm to cold for long/ or it will have a sickly life with many troubles. ¶Moreover women miscarry because of a lot of movement of their bodies and a lot of work/ and from great jumping/ especially if they jump backward after they have conceived/ as commonly occurs when dancing lewd dances of pleasure/ like the round dance. ¶Also those women who are beaten/ pushed hard/ hit/ and thrown/ and who are wont to too much unchasteness at all times miscarry easily. ¶Furthermore pregnant women also miscarry due to great anger and fear/ from shock or fright/ and sadness/ and from news of sudden joy. ¶Also when a woman miscarries her baby/ she usually has greater pain and discomfort/ than she would if she delivered naturally/ Because of the fact/ that miscarriage is against the law of nature. And the natural birth is more acceptable to and commensurate with nature.

Now here follow the signs whereby one may recognize whether a woman should or will miscarry.

¶The first sign/ when the woman's breasts/ which were healthy/ pert and firm/ and full before/ shrink/ become empty and shriveled/ or fall down/ then she will usually miscarry/ as Hippocrates and Avicenna write/ For when the woman's breasts shrink quickly and suddenly/ then she will miscarry that same day/ And if the woman is pregnant with two children/ and one breast shrivels/ which was healthy and pert before/ then she will miscarry the infant that lies on the side on which the breast has shriveled/ And Hippocrates says/ if the right breast shrivels/ then she will miscarry a boy/ since usually a boy lies on the right side/ and a girl lies on the left side. One should understand this to speak of/ a woman who is pregnant with two babies/ one a boy and one a girl. If however the babies are both boys/ or both girls/ then she will miscarry the baby that lies on the side/ which has the shriveled breast. ¶Also another sign/ when the woman feels great pain in the womb/ and her face reddens/ and her body trembles/ in fever/ with a headache/ and she feels intense pain behind her eyes against her skull/ and the woman becomes tired and has heaviness in her limbs, these signs indicate that the woman will miscarry/ in a short time from that hour/ and especially if the woman with the above signs begins to bleed heavily. ¶Also another sign/ If the woman's body swells up/

tightens and becomes hard/ but not heavy/ and the gases blow to and fro/ from one side to the other/ and especially if the gases persist/ when the woman eats or drinks things which cause gas/ This is a sign that the woman may miscarry/ due to bad gases or winds/ and especially in the second or fourth month.

How One Should Prevent and Remedy Miscarriages

¶So now the things which cause miscarriages/ and also the signs of miscarriage have been discussed. Thus it remains to be said how a woman should protect herself from miscarriage. And such protection is nothing other/ than that the woman should avoid and leave alone all the things which cause miscarriages/ which are sufficiently listed one by one above/ But in short there is something to say to this &c. First/ If the woman is concerned about miscarrying because the opening of the womb/ or genitals is too wide/ Then you should make it narrower with baths/ warming/ salves/ plasters/ and fumigations which by their nature close and tighten/ and which are spoken of above in the seventh chapter regarding the excessive bleeding and flowing which befall a woman after delivery. ¶If the woman is concerned about miscarrying because the opening of the womb is too smooth/ slippery and moist/ or the baby's cord is stopped up with slimy fluids and bad gases and winds/ then one should cure this with medicines which clean/ purge/ and dry these and consume the winds. But this should not be done without the help and advice of a wise learned doctor/ because/ there are many such fluids/ and the remedy for one is different from the remedy for another. If the woman is concerned about miscarrying due to affliction of the uterus/ or of other areas near the uterus/ such as ulcers/ boils/ abscesses/ hemorrhoids/ burning urination &c. Then one should seek advice with a doctor/ to cure such things. ¶If the woman is concerned about miscarrying because she is too thin/ dry/ and wasted/ Then she should take food and drink which moisten/ and make the body put on weight/ like good young meat/ capons/ kid/ lamb/ veal/ partridge/ and hazelhen. ¶If however the woman is concerned about miscarrying because of a serious difficult acute illness/ then one should cure the illness with the appropriate and suitable medication. ¶If the woman is concerned about miscarrying due to hunger/ then one should remedy this with appropriate food and drink/ not with gluttony. ¶If the woman is concerned about miscarrying due to excessive gluttony/ as occurs nowadays in several places/ then a suitable loss should occur. And if it is necessary/ a soft mild purgative should be used. ¶And if there is too much blood/ then a limited letting should occur to take away the blood from which the baby might suffocate in the womb. And when the pregnant woman may be let/ and when and how she may purge herself/ is described clearly and distinctly in this .viii. chapter in two consecutive items on the causes of miscarriage/ with its own foreword/ and is not necessary to repeat here. ¶If the woman is concerned about miscarrying due to heavy coughing/ vomiting/ diarrhea/ from a disease called tenasmon/ or from bleeding out of the nose or elsewhere/ Then one should remedy these things appropriately/ and have refuge with a learned doctor. ¶If the woman is concerned about miscarrying because the chorion in which the baby lies/ might easily break/ and not be able to hold the fetus because of the break/ This is difficult to prevent/ the woman must keep herself completely protected/ avoid great exercise and movement with her work/ jumping/ dancing/ running/ much standing and walking/ and lifting heavy things. ¶All other miscarriage should be prevented thus/ the woman should avoid/ flee/ shun/ and stop all things which are followed by miscarriages.

The Ninth Chapter Tells of
a Dead Baby in the Womb / Also of
the Signs of a Dead Baby / And How
One Should Bring It Out of the
Womb / By Two Methods and Ways
with Medications and Other Means

The ninth chapter tells of a dead baby in the womb. And twelve signs thereof will be described here below. The first/ is when the woman's breast becomes shriveled and soft/ as is written above in the eighth chapter on the signs of miscarriage. The second sign of a dead baby/ is when the baby no longer moves in the mother's body but had moved before. The third sign/ is when the baby falls from one side to the other like a stone/ whenever the woman turns. The fourth sign/ is when the woman's body and navel become cold/ where they had been warm before. The fifth sign/ is when evil smelly fluids come out of the uterus/ and especially if the woman has had an acute feverish illness. The sixth sign/ is when the woman's eyes sink deep into her head/ and the whites become brown/ and her ears and nose become stiff or rigid/ and her lips become lead-colored or dark blue. The seventh sign of a dead baby in the womb/ is when the woman has great pain under the navel or in the genitals/ and her face is totally misshapen and miscolored. The eighth sign/ is when the woman has a desire to eat and drink repulsive things/ different from what one normally eats and drinks. The ninth sign/ is when the woman cannot sleep. The tenth/ is when the woman has a constant burning sensation when she urinates and the desire to pass stools with much pushing and straining but little or no bowel movement. The eleventh sign/ is that the woman's breath will stink and smell evil on the second or third day after the infant is dead. The twelfth sign/ by which one can recognize if the baby is dead in the womb is/ when one lays a hand warmed in warm water on the woman's body/ if the baby does not stir due to the heat/ then it is dead. Those are twelve signs of a dead baby in the womb. And the more signs found in a pregnant woman/ the more certain it is that the baby is dead in the womb.

How One Should Bring the Dead Baby from the Womb

¶First one should take care and observe/ if one may bring the dead body from the womb/ and keep the woman alive where possible/ this is very good. Where however this is not possible/ then one should let God rule. And that the mother will not live/ should be recognized thus/ if she faints or becomes unconscious/ and becomes very forgetful or without memory/ and her limbs become very heavy and lifeless. And if she gives little or no answer when one calls her or speaks with her/ especially if she answers weakly when one calls to her in a loud voice/ and if she gets spasms/ and will not eat/ and her pulse becomes fast and light/ and if her veins tremble/ bluster and rage/ by these signs it can be recognized that one will not be able to come to the woman's aid/ nor keep her alive. Consequently one must entrust her to God. But if in fact one can bring the dead baby from the womb and keep the mother alive/ then those things just mentioned/ will not happen to her. Then one should devote oneself seriously and take great pains/ and spare no labor/ so that the woman is freed of the dead baby quickly. ¶Now one can bring a dead baby from the womb in two ways. First with medicines and without cutting and tearing the dead baby. Second/ if no medication will help/ with hooks and tongs. If you want to bring the dead baby from the womb without cutting up and dismembering the dead baby/ and also without hooks and tongs/

Then make a vapor of hooves or asses' dung/ below the woman. ¶Also another/ Make a vapor below the woman/ from a snake-skin/ myrrh/ castoreum/ yellow sulfur/ galbanum/ opopanax/ and madder/ which is used to dye things red/ and pigeon dung or hawk's dung/ One should pound all of these or their equivalent and make it all into a dough with cow bile/ and make little balls the size of hazelnuts out of it/ Lay these little balls one after another on glowing embers/ and let the smoke go up into the woman's genitals through a tube. ¶Also another/ Take thyme/ opopanax/ galbanum/ and living sulphur/ in equal amounts and mix them with cow bile/ and make little balls out of it and make a vapor/ as described above. ¶Also another/ Take one-half dram of asafetida/ three drams of dry rue/ two drams myrrh/ make a pulver out of these and mix a well-measured dram in white wine/ or in water in which savin has been boiled/ and give it to the woman to drink. ¶Also another/ Have the woman drink water/ in which figs/ fenugreek/ rue/ and dittany have been boiled/ this makes the baby slip. Then one should help it from its place with the above-named things. ¶Also another/ Take gum ammoniac/ opopanax/ christmas rose called elleborus in Latin/ stavesacre/ called staphisagria in Latin/ and birthwort/ in Latin Aristologia longa/ and colocynth without the seeds. Pulverize all these things/ and mix them with cow bile and with green rue juice/ and make a plug with cotton wool or other wool/ coat the plug well/ and make it very moist in the same juice and cow bile/ and shove it in the woman's genitals. ¶Also another/ Make a little plug out of cotton/ the length/ and size of the middle finger/ and moisten it in rue juice/ in which scammony has been mixed/ and shove the little plug in the woman's genitals. ¶Also another/ Take equal amounts of well-pulverized round birthwort/ savin/ and watercress and mix them with cow bile and moisten in this a little plug the same size and length as above/ and use it as described above. ¶Also another/ The woman should drink the milk of another woman/ then the dead baby will come out of her. ¶Also take dittany juice or a powder of its roots in the weight of .ii. drams/ and give it to the woman to drink in wine/ if she does not have high fever/

or give it to her in warm water/ if she has fever/ this drives the baby out harmlessly. ¶Also another/ Take .i. lot myrrh/ .ii. drams each/ cinnamon sticks/ galbanum/ and castoreum/ .i. dram opopanax. Mix these things with cow bile/ make a pill out of it weighing .i. dram/ and lay it on glowing coal and let the steam go up into the woman's genitals. This steam drives out the dead baby/ and the inflammation/ and also the suffocation of blood from the woman. ¶Also a bath in addition/ take a handful each of water mint/ southernwood/ mugwort/ .i. lot bitumen/ .v. lots madder/ .iiii. lots each camomile blossoms/ blind nettles/ and fenugreek/ Boil all these things in rain water/ and the woman should bathe in it/ then take one lot each of chicken fat and duck fat/ and .iiii. lots of dill oil/ rub her skin with this when she comes out of the bath/ then give her one and one-half drams of powdered date kernels/ and one-third of a dram of saffron/ to drink in white wine. ¶Also another/ Take opopanax/ make a little plug out of it like a finger/ the woman should shove this in her genitals/ for it pulls the dead baby out. ¶Also another/ Take a dram or a little less of galbanum/ and three or four lots of goats' milk/ stir the galbanum into the milk and give it to the woman to drink. ¶Also another/ Take galbanum and stir it into mugwort juice and make a plaster out of it with a little wax and spread it on a cloth a knife's thickness/ long and wide enough so that it can reach from the right side to the left side/ and from the navel to the genitals. ¶Also another/ Take treacle which is called diatesseron in Latin and give it to the woman/ it drives out the dead baby. ¶And if all such medicines and things which are described in succession above will not drive out the dead baby/ then one must look seriously at the situation and bring the dead baby from the mother with hooks/ iron tongs/ and other tools made for this/ and one should do this as follows/ One should lay the woman on her back/ with the head very low and the legs high above her/ and should hold the woman strong and tight by the arms on both sides and tie her fast/ so that one does not pull her closer when one pulls the baby out. Then the midwife should open the woman's privates with the left hand salved with white-lily oil or with other things that make it smooth and slippery/ so that the fingers are well coated and covered. And she should reach into the woman's privates and seek the limbs of the dead baby/ so that she knows where to begin with the iron hook/ and may thus pull out the dead baby. Now if the dead baby lays in the womb with the head toward the birth canal then the midwife should drive the hook into one of the baby's eyes/ or in the roof of the mouth/ or under the chin in the neck/ or in a shoulder blade/ or in other limbs of the baby into which the hook will go. If however the baby presents itself with its feet toward the birth canal then the midwife should drive the hook into the bones above the baby's genitals like the middle rib or into the breast bone/ or behind into the back. When she has driven in a hook then she should hold it with her right hand/ but not pull yet/ and with her left hand she should reach inside the woman and push another hook into the dead baby opposite the first hook. Then the midwife should slowly pull with both hands at once/ and not with one alone/ so that the dead baby is pulled from both sides equally. And she should pull slowly/ and not straight out/ but rather from one side to the other/ and as she gently pulls she should reach into the woman with a well-oiled index finger and free and loosen the baby all around from the mother/ and skillfully bring it to the opening/ and peel it away if it is attached. If the dead baby will move from its place through such pulling the midwife should push the hooks longer and higher into the baby, if necessary, until the baby is completely pulled out of the mother's body. And if it happens that one hand of the dead baby appears alone without the other and one cannot easily shove it back into the womb/ due to the narrowness of the opening of the uterus/ Then one should bind a cloth around the baby's hand so that it will not move or slip away/ and should pull on the hand until the arm comes completely out/ then one should cut off the arm at the armpit. One should do the same thing if both hands and arms of the dead baby appear alone up to the elbows/ or with other parts if one cannot bring them back to their proper place/ for example if one or both feet appear in the birth canal and the body will not follow/ Then one should pull out the legs and cut them off up near the genitals in the same way. The surgeons should have special instruments and tools for this/ like scissors/ iron tongs and iron hooks/ with which such things can be quickly/ easily and lightly pulled out and cut. Then she should bind/ shove and pull what is left of the dead baby whether it is whole or in pieces/ until the dead infant comes completely out of the mother. ¶And if the dead baby's head is so big from being puffed up and swollen or full of evil moisture and fluids/ that it cannot come out of the womb due to the narrowness of the opening/ Then the midwife should take a lancet or a small sharp knife between her fingers/ and she should open up the dead baby's head/ this will make the head smaller/ as the fluids and water flow out of the head. And if the head is naturally too big/ then the midwife should break up/ crush/ split/ and divide the head as she may/ and pull out the pieces of the skull with tongs used for extracting teeth. ¶Further if the head is removed from the womb/ and the dead baby's breast will not follow due to its size/ or the narrowness of the opening/ then one should crush and split the breast as one may and lift it near the shoulder blade/ so that it will move from its place. The same if the dead baby's body is swollen and puffed up/ then one should cut open the body/ so that it shrinks and becomes smaller/ and the waters flow out. ¶And if it happens that at the time there is a dead baby in the womb/ the entrance to the uterus is too narrow due to swelling and too dry due to acute ulcers or boils/ then one should not take it upon oneself to bring the dead baby from her before one has made a suitable and wide exit for the baby/ with fatty oils and smooth fats/ and with sitting in a bath of water/ or with warming of the uterus. And if after the delivery of the dead baby the woman has too much blood flowing/ then one should help her as described above in the .vii. chapter on the conditions of a woman after a natural delivery. ¶Also if the baby presents one side in the birth canal/ if it is possible/ then one should arrange and shove it to the proper delivery. Then one should warm/ salve and smear the uterus/ so that the uterus is widened. If however the dead baby will not allow itself to be shoved/ then one should cut it to pieces inside/ as stated above. ¶Furthermore if it happens that the mother is dead which one can recognize through signs of a dead person/ and if there is still a hope that the baby lives/ Then you should hold the woman's mouth/ uterus/ and genitals open/ so that the baby has air and breath/ as women usually know. Then you should cut open the dead women along the length of the left side with a razor/ for the left side is freer and emptier than the right side/ this is because the liver lies in the right side. And when you cut open the woman/ then reach in with your hands and pull the baby out/ Thus we read in Roman history/ that the first emperor called Julius/ was cut out of his mother's womb/ And so it is called Caesar/ after one who has been much spoken of as having been cut from the womb.*

*The German here is confusing: "Darumb heißt er Cesar/ dz als vyl gesprochen ist als ein ußgeschnitner von muter leib." Working from the Latin in 1540, Richard Jonas translates this as "and they that are borne after this fashion be called Cesares, for because they be cut out of their mother's belly, whereupon also the noble Roman Cesar the 1st of that name in Rome toke his name" (Richard Jonas, The Byrth of Mankynde, 1540).

The Tenth Chapter
Tells How One
Should Handle / Protect /
And Look After the Newborn Baby /
Also How One Should Take Care of It

When the baby has been born/ one should cut its navel four finger widths from its body and tie it/ as Avicenna writes. And on the cut one should lay a mild pulver of bolus armenus and dragon's blood/ sarcocolla*/ myrrh and roman caraway all in equal amounts/ and then one should lay cotton soaked in olive oil on the pulver/ and then bind it so that it does not fall off. But some doctors say one should tie the navel three finger widths from the baby's body/ and then cut it. Moreover it is said that if the navel of a boy is cut long or short/ then his tongue will be long or short accordingly. ¶Furthermore Avicenna also writes of the navel/ When a woman delivers her first baby/ then one should examine the baby's navel at the place where it touches the baby's body/ and if at that place the navel is not wrinkled or knobby/ then that woman will not have any more children after this child. If there are wrinkles or knobs on it/ then after this child she will have as many children as there are wrinkles or knobs on the navel. Other doctors also write the same and more/ If the wrinkles lay far from each other/ then there will be a long time between the children which will be born. If they lay close to each other/ then there will be a short time between those children which will be born. And black or red wrinkles mean

*Sarcocol gum.

boys/ and white ones girls. ¶Also one should salve and smear the baby with oil made from acorns/ this oil makes the baby's skin firm and fit/ so that the outside things that touch the baby/ don't hurt or injure it/ For after the child has been born everything that touches it is unpleasant/ raw and cold to it. Also one should bathe the baby in lukewarm water. And one should gently clean its nostrils well with fingers/ with cut nails. One should also drop a little olive oil into its eyes. Also the mother or the nurse should touch it on the anus/ so that it is inclined and stimulated to pass stools/ and one should keep it warm and protect it from the cold. And when the navel falls off/ this usually happens after three or four days/ then one should lay on its navel ash and fish shells which one finds in ponds/ or ashes from calves' hooves or bream ash well pulverized and mixed with wine. And when you want to swaddle the baby/ then you should softly take hold of and touch its limbs/ stretch each limb/ arrange/ and order them as they should be/ and such swaddling should occur often. One should dry its eyes often and frequently with a soft silk or linen cloth. One should also softly stroke it over the bladder/ so that its urinating becomes easier. One should also stretch its arms and arrange them at its sides down by its knees. One should place a little cap on its head/ and lay it to bed at the end of the house where it is not too cold. One should make it a little dark for it and give it shade/ so that the light of the sun does not shine on it, and when you lay it to sleep/ you should lay the head much higher than the body/ and ensure that it is not pressed or placed crooked at the neck/ at the back/ or other limbs. And if it is summer/ then it should be bathed in lukewarm water and in winter in warm water/ although not so that it burns. One should wash it two or three times each day/ always when it has had a good sleep. One should not bathe it any longer than until its body becomes red and warm. One should also prevent any water from going into the baby's ears. Afterward when you take the baby out of the bath/ you should dry it with soft cloths/ and lay it in the nurse's lap/ and wrap up its back as is custom/ and drip one or two drops of good olive oil in its nostrils/ this is good for the sight.

The Eleventh Chapter
Tells How One
Should Nurse a Baby /
And How Long and How the
Wet-Nurse and Her Milk Should Be &c.

As much as the mother may/ she should nurse her own baby and not give it to another woman/ For the mother's milk is suitable/ proper/ and appropriate for the baby/ and gives it much nourishment/ considering that it is the same as the nourishment that the baby had in the womb. The baby is also much more willing and eager to suckle its own mother's milk. For as Avicenna says/ the milk of its mother is also healthier for it and it is enough/ when it suckles two or three times a day/ But at first one should not overfeed the baby/ or feed it too much at one time/ Because it is better to nurse it a little/ and more frequently/ a little at a time/ and after a short while a little more/ For if one overnurses and overfeeds the baby at one time/ then its body stretches/ and swells/ and it gets a lot of wind in it/ and its urine becomes white/ this comes from indigestion of the extra milk. And if this happens to the baby/ then one should not nurse it for a long time until it is very hungry. And if the woman has sharp or bitter milk then she should not nurse the baby on an empty stomach. ¶If however the mother does not wish or want to nurse the baby herself/ because of illness/ or because her milk is bad/ Then one may give the baby to a wet-nurse/ But the wet-nurse should have the qualities that are written below. First the wet-nurse should have good color/ a strong throat/ and a strong wide bosom. Second she should not be too close to her delivery/

nor too far from it/ and at least one and one-half or two months should have passed since her delivery/ and this wet-nurse should have delivered a boy. Third the wet-nurse should have a healthy body/ neither too thin nor too fat so that she has a firm/ hard/ fleshy body. Fourth the wet-nurse should have good conduct and demeanor/ not easily falling into anger/ sadness and fear/ For bad conduct, demeanor, and anger &c. are damaging to the baby/ and make the milk bad. For this reason one should not let shrews and dumb women nurse babies. Fifth/ the wet-nurse's breasts should be firm and full/ not empty/ loose or soft/ neither too big nor too small/ and not too hard. Sixth the nurse's milk should not be brown/ nor green/ nor yellow/ nor red/ nor bitter/ nor salty/ and not too coarse or thick. And the best milk is tried and proved thus/ When you spray a little on the nail of your thumb and tilt your thumb/ if the milk does not flow or run down then it is too coarse and thick. If you do not tilt your thumb down/ and the milk flows and runs down anyway then the milk is too thin runny and watery/ It follows from this/ that the best milk is that which does not flow or run off of an untilted thumb/ but which easily flows and runs when you tilt your thumb/ This milk is appropriately blended/ and properly mixed/ neither too thick nor too thin. ¶Further if the milk is too hot/ then the wet-nurse should not nurse the baby on an empty stomach. Also if there is too little milk/ this occurs due to illness of the whole body/ or from illness of the breast. Moreover it also comes from congestion or cold in the breast or because the breast out of which milk should come is not pulled enough/ Also because the wet-nurse has a lack of food or drink. In order to really recognize and remedy these causes/ As Avicenna writes/ one should resort to the learned doctors/ and seek advice from them. But to give some comfort to those women/ whose milk is lacking/ Note here that using the seeds from pastinaca/ parsnip in English and also the root of that plant increases the woman's milk. ¶Also another which increases the milk in the woman's breast. The woman should eat and enjoy a broth of barley/ chickpeas/ gray peas/ and in this same broth she should boil fennel root or seeds. ¶Also she should eat sheep's udder with the milk that is in it. ¶Also another/ The woman should drink barley water with a dram of dried powdered earthworms. ¶Also another/ Take dairy butter and stir two lots of it in wine and give it to her to drink. ¶Also another/ The woman should set a cupping glass under her breast without pricking or cutting. ¶Also another/ The woman should lay under or on her breast a plaster made of frankincense/ mastic/ and pitch/ but one should rub her body beforehand with olive oil/ so that it does not stick fast. ¶Also the woman should softly rub her breast/ or let it soak a little in a warm bath after eating. ¶Also the woman should warm her breast with wool soaked in white-lily oil/ or violet oil/ in which musk/ frankincense/ and laudanum have been stirred. Or she should warm her breast with good wine/ in which mint/ roses/ violets/ and a wood called aloes have been boiled. ¶Also another/ The woman should eat good meat/ good broth made with cinnamon stick/ mace/ cardamon/ and with egg yolks. She should also eat milk and new cheese/ and she should also not overwork. ¶Also another thing to increase the milk. The woman should eat good pap made with bean flour/ rice/ and dry white bread with milk and sugar/ and it would be good if she adds a little fennel seed to it. ¶Also another/ Take three drams each/ of anise and siler montan/ and one-half lot of crystal/ make these into a good pulver/ and add twice as much sugar to it/ give this to the woman with white wine eight or ten times/ in the morning/ midday/ and at night. ¶Also another/ Take a handful each of fennel seeds or herb/ and horehound/ Two lots of aniseed and one-third of a dram of powdered saffron/ and six lots of fresh butter/ and boil these with just enough water/ and make a plaster on the woman's breast/ and lay it on warm. ¶Also another/ Take three lots of well-pounded roman caraway and boil it in four pounds of water/ with six lots of purified honey in a new pot until it is reduced by one-third/ she should drink this water often. ¶Also another/ Take two lots of well-washed cabbage/ and one lot roman caraway/ twelve lots honey/ pound the cabbage and caraway well/ and make an electuary with the honey/ the woman should take a spoonful of this electuary when she goes to sleep/ and also in the morning on an empty stomach. ¶Also another/ Take one lot of well-pulverized crystal/ separate the powder in four parts/ the woman should take this same powder on an empty stomach four mornings in a row/ each time with a broth of chickpeas or red peas. ¶Also these things increase the milk/ dill weed and its seeds/ aniseed/ horehound/ cardamom/ new cheese and old whey/ chickpeas/ crystal powdered and given with honey/ lettuce made into a salad/ fennel seeds/ wine in which rosemary has been boiled/ or wild pennyroyal that is wild thyme/ or houseleek. ¶Furthermore the wet nurse should not be unchaste/ because this decreases the milk and makes it distasteful and unpleasant for the baby/ because of this the baby rarely keeps the milk down. ¶Also it is good if the baby does not nurse from its own mother on the first day/ but rather from another woman. And if the wet-nurse becomes sick or has dysentery or is tight and constipated/ or has taken strong medicines to bring on defecation/ then it is better for another woman to nurse the baby. ¶Furthermore if the baby has nursed and one is laying it to sleep/ then one should rock it slowly/ so that the milk does not go back and forth/ and move/ and become unclean and bad. ¶Furthermore Avicenna says that according to nature one should nurse a baby for two years/ although this is against the custom practiced now. ¶Furthermore one should not wean the baby from the milk abruptly. One should make round plugs of bread and sugar/ so that it becomes used to eating coarse foods. There is much more learning and instruction about babies and how one should hold and handle them, in particular when their teeth begin to grow and come out/ Avicenna writes of this/ and it is not necessary to write of it here.

The Twelfth Chapter Tells of Various
Conditions and Diseases of the Newborn Baby / And How One Should Come to Their Aid

Since the diseases and conditions which befit a newborn baby are many/ As say Hippocrates/ Galen/ Rhazes/ Avicenna/ Averroes/ and other doctors/ to write all of them here would be slow and also tiresome. Because of this here will be written only the most notable diseases and conditions which befall the newborn baby/ ordered in succession. And with this the twelfth chapter/ and this entire book will be completed. And here are the diseases which will be described in succession.

New-born babies have the following diseases or conditions

Boils or ulcers.
Dysentery or diarrhea.
Constipation of the stools.
Spasms.
Heavy coughing.
Short breath.
Sores on the tongue.
Tears on the mouth.
Fluid in the ears.
A hot abscess of the brain.
Swelling of the eyes.
Miscoloring of the eyes.
Unnaturally high heat.
Sickness in the body.
Swelling of the body.
Too much sneezing.
Sores on the body.
Swelling of the genitals.
Swelling of the navel.
Lack of sleep.
Belching or hiccups.
Vomiting or throwing up.
Nightmares.
Proneness to falling sickness.

100

A rasping breath.

Protrusion of the rectum.

Tenasmon.*

Worms in the anus.

Soreness of the skin.

Falling sickness.

Excessive thinness.

Wasting of the body.

Lameness of the baby.

Trembling of the limbs.

Stone in the bladder.

Squinting in the eyes.

Boils or Ulcers

¶If the baby has boils or ulcers/ or abscesses in the gums where the teeth grow/ or in the gums of the jaw bone/ then one should softly rub or press it on the gums and the boils with the fingers/ and rub and salve it well with chicken fat/ hare's brain/ and camomile oil mixed with honey or with turpentine that is mixed with honey. And one should pour warm water in which camomile blossoms and dill have been boiled down onto its head from a height of two spans.

On Dysentery or Diarrhea

¶Moreover if the baby gets dysentery or diarrhea/ then one should make a plaster on its body of rose seeds/ roman caraway/ and anise or apple seeds. If this will not help/ then give it as much as one-sixth part of a dram or a little more of rennet from a kid/ with cold water/ and that day one should not give it any milk/ so that the milk does not run into the baby's stomach/ but one should give it a soft-boiled egg yolk/ or white bread cooked in water/ or a thin wheat flour pap cooked in water. ¶Furthermore if the baby's stool is yellow/ then one should give it rose syrup/ or syrup from sour crab apples/ or pomegranate syrup with a little mint water. ¶Also take yeast and blend it in water/ and sieve it through a cloth/ and take the sixth part of a dram of violet and one-third of a dram of burned elephant bone called spodium in Latin/ and one and one-half drams of oak apple/ and

*Tenesmus.

give it to the baby to drink. ¶Also another/ Take burdock seeds/ pound them and mix them with a roasted egg yolk and give it to the baby to eat. ¶Also another/ Take pounded oak apples/ boil the powder in water/ and with this water and barley flour or millet flour make a plaster and lay it on the baby's body. And if that will not help/ then take a dram each of sloe juice called accacia in Latin/ and white lead/ and the sixth part of a dram of opium/ and one dram of sugar/ make a little plug out of this one and one-half fingers long and in the thickness of a quill/ and shove it in the baby's behind/ it disappears. ¶Further if the stools are white/ then one should give the baby one-eighth of a dram of the confection gallia muscata with quince juice and one-third of a dram of frankincense. ¶Also another/ Take one part saffron/ three parts myrrh/ mix these with red wine and lay it on the baby's body. ¶Also another/ Take knotgrass juice and egg whites/ and mix them with rose powder and bloodstone called ematites in Latin/ and with mastic/ incense/ a red earth called bolo armeno/ dragon's blood/ and pomegranate rinds/ make a plaster out of these and lay it on the baby's body. ¶Also another/ Boil rose leaves in water and bathe the baby in it. ¶Also another/ Take two parts comfrey juice/ one part each broad-leaved plantain juice and lance-leaved plantain juice/ stir into this juice roasted clay from an oven/ and make a plaster of this and lay it on the baby's body.

On Constipation of the Stools

And if the newborn baby becomes compact and hard in its body and is not able to pass its stools/ then you should make a little suppository for it/ as big and wide as a quill pen/ and half a finger long/ out of honey boiled until it becomes hard/ and you should moisten this in oil/ and shove it in the baby's behind/ or make a little plug from sorrel or from iris root/ in the same size and length and moistened in oil as above. ¶Also another/ Give it a little honey to eat, the size of a chickpea/ also you should softly rub its body with cotton moistened in oil/ or lay cow's bile or ox bile in cotton or other wool on its navel. ¶Also another/

Give the wet-nurse a medicine which brings on bowel move-
ments/ then the second day after she should nurse the baby.
¶Also another/ Take one-half dram of nutmeg and pound it
with the fat from a ram's kidneys/ and make a little plug out of
it in the size and length as described above and shove it in the
baby's bottom. ¶Also another/ Take a handful each of mallow
and althea leaves/ a handful each of fenugreek seeds and lin-
seeds/ and four lots of althea root/ ten figs/ boil all these well in
water/ then pound them well in a stone so that it becomes like
a porridge or pap and add four lots of butter to it and four lots
of chicken fat/ and one-third of a dram of saffron. Make a
plaster out of this and spread it on a cloth to the thickness of a
quill pen/ and lay it warm on the baby's body day and night/
then if the baby still does not pass a stool lay this on it afterward/
Take a dram of aloe/ the fourth part of a dram each of white
hellebore and black hellebore/ pound these well to a powder and
take three tablespoons full of dwarf elder juice or ox bile and mix
the above things with it/ and moisten wool in this and lay it the
width of a hand on the baby's navel. ¶Also another/ Take dwarf
elder juice and flour dust and make a porridge out of it in a pan
and spread it on a cloth to the thickness of a quill pen/ and lay
it warm the width of a hand on the baby's navel/ and under the
navel/ but not on its stomach. Also boil two handfuls of rose
leaves in a little sack that is four fingers wide/ in the quenching
water from the blacksmith/ with a little vinegar/ dry the little
sack well and lay it warm on the baby's stomach. ¶Also another/
Take butter and put it in a nutshell and bind it on the navel.
One should also rub and smear its body with butter.

For Convulsions or Cramps

And if at the time its teeth come the baby gets a sickness
which is called spasmus in Latin/ this is usually caused by indigestion and from nervous instability/ and such a disease occurs particularly in fat babies/ then you should salve it with
blue-lily oil/ or white-lily oil/ or with yellow–clove blossom oil/

called oleum de keyri in Latin. ¶Furthermore if the baby gets a cramp or spasm so that its limbs stick out from it then you should bathe it in water/ in which mullein/ which is also called candlewick/ has been boiled/ or salve it with violet oil/ and sweet almond oil/ mixed together. And if the heat is very great/ then salve it with olive oil alone/ or with violet oil mixed with a little white wax and apply violet oil to its head.

For Heavy Coughs

¶Furthermore if the baby coughs a lot/ and the fluids from its head fall/ in its nose/ in its mouth/ and on its chest/ Then you should pour warm water on its head from a height of two spans for one-half hour without interruption/ and salve its tongue with honey/ After this softly take hold of its tongue in the back of its mouth and push it back a little/ so that a lot of phlegm breaks from it/ then it will become healthy. Or take gum arabic/ and gum tragacanth/ quince seeds and licorice juice/ and sugar penids*/ pound them all together and give a little to the baby each day with newly drawn milk. ¶Also another/ Take shelled sweet almonds and pound them together well/ and boil them in fennel juice or water and give it to the baby in the evening and morning. Or take fennel water/ mix it with milk and give it to the baby. And if the baby's tongue and gums are raw and dry from coughing/ then take two spoonfuls of coarsely pounded quince seeds and lay them for two or three hours in six spoonfuls of warm water/ then push the slime from this through a cloth and put it in a little pan with sugar penids/ and with a little sweet almond oil/ make a thin electuary out of it/ and give it to the baby often. And if the baby also has a high fever with its cough/

---

*Sugar penids "are prepared of sugar dissolved in spring water by a gentle fire, and the whites of eggs diligently beaten, and clarified once, and again whilst it is boyling, then strain it and boyl it gently again, til it rise up in great bubles, and being chewed it stick not to your teeth, then powr it upon a marble, anointed with Oyl of Almonds . . . bring back the outsides of it to the middle til it look like larch Rozin, then your hands being rubbed with white starch, you may draw it into threads" (Culpepper, p. 221).

then add sweet pomegranate juice to the electuary. ¶Also another/ If the baby has a cough with fever then take one-half lot each of white poppy seeds/ and gum tragacanth/ one lot of shelled pumpkin seeds/ pound these things well/ mix it with water in which big raisins or grapes or a fruit called sebestens have been boiled/ And give it often to the baby to eat. ¶Also another/ Take raisins or grapes without the seeds/ and boil them in water in an iron pan/ but do not let them burn/ then take them from the fire/ and pound them very well in a stone/ and add an equal amount of sugar penids to it/ give an amount the size of an olive stone to the baby early and late. ¶Also if the baby's cough comes from cold things/ then take a little powdered or pounded myrrh/ and mix it with boiled honey/ and with a little sweet almond oil and give it to the baby. ¶Also the wet-nurse should avoid all things that cause coughs/ like vinegar/ salty foods/ pungent things/ nuts/ and she should salve and smear her breast with butter and dyaltea. ¶Also an excellent cure for a baby's cough. Take wine grapes or raisins separated from the seeds/ and roast them dry in a hot little pan/ then mix it together and add an equal amount of sugar penids to it/ with a little violet oil/ and make a soft electuary/ give an amount the size of a hazelnut to the baby often.

For a Short Tight Breath

¶Also for tightness and shortness of breath in the baby pulverize linseeds/ and mix them with honey and give it to the baby often. And if the baby becomes tight-chested and is overcome by shortness of breath/ then you should salve and smear it well around and behind the ears with olive oil/ do the same to the tongue/ so that it vomits/ and drip warm water in its mouth/ and give it a little pounded linseed/ mixed with honey as an electuary. ¶Also another/ Take cotton seeds or kernels which you find in cotton/ and give it to the baby powdered in a cooked egg yolk. ¶Also another/ If the baby has a tight hard breath with diarrhea/ then give it siripum mirtinum/ boiled in milk/ or give it date kernels boiled with rye flour and milk.

Sores on the Tongue

¶It also happens to little babies/ that many small sores grow on the tongue and in the mouth/ this comes from sharpness which is in the mother's milk/ for the baby's tongue and mouth are so delicate/ soft and tender that they become torn through touching. Consequently they become even more torn from the sharpness of the milk/ and when such a thing befalls a baby then it hurts it a great deal/ and if the sores become black and are gangrenous/ then they are evil and deadly to the baby. But those that are white and yellow are less evil. And to counter such sores take pounded violets and lay them in its mouth. Or take violets/ roses/ and carob bean called xilocaracta in Latin/ pound them together and lay it on the baby's sores. ¶Also take lettuce juice and nightshade and purslane juice/ mix them together and spread it on the baby's sores. And if the sores are black and gangrenous/ then pound licorice and add it to the above juices. ¶Also if the blisters are wet/ then you should take myrrh/ oak apple/ and frankincense rinds well powdered/ mix these with honey and spread it on the tongue. ¶Also another/ Take the juice of sour mulberries or the juice from unripe wine grapes/ and spread it on the tongue. It is also good to wash the sores with wine/ and then spread oak-apple powder or frankincense rinds on them. ¶If you want to use something stronger/ take .iii. drams each of bolus armenus/ and the rinds of pomegranates/ and sumac/ and .ii. drams oak apples/ and .i. dram alum/ grind these things finely/ push them through a sieve and lay the powder on the blisters. ¶Also if the baby has sores in the mouth which are red and cause great pain and a lot of saliva/ Then the wet-nurse should eat cold and moist food/ then she should chew lentils well/ and lay them in the baby's mouth. Or take starch or cornstarch and blend it in rose water and lay it on the baby's tongue/ or lay the juice from pomegranate or quince or crab apple in the baby's mouth. ¶Also if the blisters are yellow/ then mix the following juices/ lettuce juice/ purslane juice. But if the blisters are white/ then take a dram each of myrrh and saffron and two drams of white sugar/ make a powder of them/ and lay it on the baby's tongue.

On Chapped Mouth

¶Further if the baby's mouth breaks out or becomes cracked or torn/ this usually occurs due to hardness of the wet-nurse's nipples/ then take pulled or carded cotton/ and lay it in broad-leaved or lance-leaved plantain juice/ or in unrefined butter/ or in fresh chicken fat/ and warm it all and rub the inside of the baby's mouth/ and in particular rub the lips with the cotton moistened in these warm things.

On Fluid in the Ears

¶Further it also befalls babies that their ears run and flow/ and this comes from excessive moisture in the body/ and in particular in the head. You should help this as follows/ Take wool and moisten it in honey mixed with red wine and with a little powdered alum/ or with a little saffron/ and then make a little plug or pledget out of the wool/ and put it in its ear/ and when the wool becomes full of foulness and fluids then pull it out of the baby's ear/ then take boiled honey/ temper it with water/ and put it in the ear. Or take pounded oak apples and mix them with vinegar and put it in. ¶Further if the baby has an earache from the wind or from gases and moisture/ then you should boil dittany or myrrh in olive oil/ and drip it lukewarm into its ear.

A Hot Abscess of the Brain*

¶When the baby gets a hot abscess of the brain/ so that its throat or eyes hurt/ and its face becomes pale or yellow/ then you should make its head cool and moist as follows. Take pumpkin/ nightshade and purslane juice/ mix them with rose oil and moisten cotton in it/ and lay it on its head/ and when the cotton becomes dry/ lay a fresh one on.

*In Avicenna this is listed under "Meningitis" (Avicenna, p. 294).

Swelling of the Eyes*

¶When the baby has swelling of the eyes/ then take a juice called licium and mix it with woman's milk/ and lay it on the eyes with soft cloths. Then wash its eyes with water in which camomile blossoms and basil have been boiled. But if the eyes are not red with the swelling/ nor the forehead heated/ then take myrrh/ saffron/ aloe/ and rose leaves/ mix all these things with good wine/ and lay it with a little cloth on the eyes/ and put a little amber mixed with woman's milk in its nostrils.

Miscoloring of the Eyes

¶Furthermore if from much crying the baby's eyes become white/ Then put nightshade juice in its eyes. And if the baby's eyelids become red/ shabby/ scabby/ and swollen from much crying/ then salve the veins with nightshade juice.

Unnaturally High Heat

¶When the baby gets an unnaturally high heat which is called febris in Latin/ then the wet-nurse or nursing mother should eat and drink things that cool and moisten. Also one should give the baby juice from pomegranate/ and give it pumpkin water with sugar and with a little camphor to drink. Then it would be good to make it sweat. ¶Also another/ Take barley flour and mix it with wormwood juice and with plantain/ mallows/ and with houseleek/ and make a plaster and lay it on the baby's chest. ¶Also another/ Salve or smear the baby with rose oil/ and violet oil mixed with poplar buds on the brow/ on the temples/ and on the arms down by the hands/ on the veins/ and down on the feet at the ankles. Spread this salve on cold. ¶Also

---

*"Conjunctivitis" (Avicenna, p. 295).

another/ Make a plaster for it with barley flour and dried pulverized roses/ mix both of these with rose water and with sow thistle tea and when you bathe the baby/ you should bathe it in water in which herbs of a cold nature have been boiled/ like lettuce, purslane, sow thistle, liverwort, and plantain.

Sickness in the Body*

¶And if the baby's stomach hurts and it cries and squirms/ then you should lay cotton moistened in warm water and warm oil with a little wax on its stomach.

Swelling in the Body

¶And if the baby has swelling all over its body or in some of its limbs/ then take black elder shoots/ and dwarf elder shoots/ and boil them in white wine/ and wrap the baby in it/ and take care that it does not get hot. And if the baby's stomach becomes swollen accompanied by a strong headache/ then take myrrh/ aloe epaticum and saffron/ temper these with bean juice and lay it on its head.

Too Much Sneezing

¶Furthermore if the baby sneezes too much/ and it is due to an abscess of the brain/ then you should lay things that cool on the baby's head/ be they salves/ oils/ juices/ or other. If the sneezing does not come from an abscess/ then pound either green or dry basil and put it in the baby's nose. And if the sneezing comes with heat/ and the baby's eyes are sunk deep/ then lay purslane leaves on its head, or take thinly scraped pumpkin/ mix it with rose oil and barley flour and lay it on its head with egg yolks and rose oil.

*Colic.

Sores on the Body

¶If the baby's body is covered with sores/ and they are black and full of pus then this is deadly, and it is even more deadly if there are many sores. But if the sores are white/ then the baby may well recover, the same if they are red. For this take rose leaves/ and leaves from an herb called myrtle/ and tamarisk/ boil these things in water/ in the same water moisten cloths and lay these on the baby's sores. ¶Also salve it with rose oil/ with myrtle oil/ with tamarisk oil. And if the sores are white or red/ then let them ripen/ then they will heal. But if they fester and open then make a salve from white lead/ which is called ungentum de cerusa in Latin which you find in the apothecary/ you should salve the sores with this. ¶Also another/ It is also good/ to wash the sores with honey water/ in which a salt called in Latin nitrum* has been stirred. Avicenna writes more on this/ and if it is necessary then seek further advice from the learned doctors.

On Swelling Near the Genitals

¶Also if it happens that from too much crying/ the baby swells or spreads near the genitals in the joints/ Then take a seed called ameos† well pounded and mix it with egg white and lay it on the swelling or spreading/ and bind it to with a soft clean silk or linen cloth. Or take roasted bitter lupines/ which are called lupini amari in Latin/ and lay them in wine/ and add myrrh to it/ and boil them both in wine/ make a plaster out of it and lay it on the aby's swelling. ¶Also another plaster to put on swelling of babies. Take .xv. drams of alum/ .ii. drams of oak apples/ pound them well and boil them in red wine until it becomes thick/ and lay it on the swelling/ and lay a soft bath sponge on it/ moistened with vinegar mixed with water/ and when it falls

*Saltpeter.
†Bishop's weed.

off then lay another on it. ¶Also another/ Spread leather sizing on a cloth and lay it on the swelling and bind it/ and when it falls off then lay another on.

On Swelling of the Navel

¶When it happens that there is swelling in the baby's navel/ and especially where the navel is cut/ then help it as follows. Take spica/ which you put in lye/ called "Mary magdalene blossoms" in German*/ turpentine/ and an oil from sesames/ boil all these together/ moisten cotton in it and lay it on the baby's navel a thumb thick. ¶Also another/ If the baby's navel swells from much crying or heavy coughing/ or from falling or hitting/ Then take lupines/ and clean old cloths/ and burn them so that they become like tinder/ pound them to a pulver/ mix them with red wine/ and spread it on hemp/ and lay it on the baby's navel.

Decrease in Natural Sleep

¶Furthermore if the baby will not sleep/ and cries without cease/ then make it sleep as follows. Take the stems of poppies/ or the hulls from the heads/ and also the poppy seeds/ and lettuce oil/ and poppy seed oil/ temper these things together and lay it on the baby's brow and temples with soft cloths/ this helps greatly. ¶Also if the nursing baby will not sleep due to impurity of the milk it suckles then help it thus. Take violet oil/ with a little vinegar and put it often in its nostrils. Or take rose oil mixed with lettuce juice/ and salve its head and also its stomach with this/ and be sure that the wet-nurse's milk is good. And give the baby a syrup of white poppy seeds to suck/ and salve its brow and temples with violet oil in which a little saffron and opium have been stirred.

*Avicenna recommends "celtic juice and turpentine resin melted in sesame oil" (Avicenna, p. 296).

On Belching or Hiccups

¶When the baby has hiccups/ then take a nut called nux indica* in Latin/ Pound it and mix it with sugar and give it to the baby to eat. ¶Also sometimes belches come to the baby from overfullness/ or from hunger and emptiness of the stomach/ if it comes from overfullness/ or from a coldness of the stomach/ then salve or smear its stomach with warm laurel oil/ or make a plaster with powdered dill seeds mixed with mint juice/ and lay it warm on its stomach/ but if the belching comes from an empty or hungry stomach/ then take violet oil or rose oil/ or milk thistle juice/ or a juice from other cold herbs/ mix these things with mother's milk/ and salve its stomach as described above. Also give it milk to drink or another good drink. And if the baby vomits this up/ still enough will remain to keep its stomach moist.

On Vomiting

¶Vomiting also occurs in a baby/ for this you should give it four barley corns' weight of ground cloves. ¶Also make a plaster for the esophagus/ Take mastic/ frankincense and dried rose leaves/ and pulverize them all/ and temper them with mint juice/ and if there is much belching add a little vinegar to it. ¶Also another/ Take white wheat flour/ and roast it until it becomes red/ and put it in vinegar and grind it fine/ and add hard egg yolks to it/ and a little mastic/ frankincense/ and gum arabic/ temper these with mint juice and make a plaster out of them/ lay it on the esophagus/ and hold a warm toast of bread in front of its mouth and nose. ¶Also the nursing baby can be stricken with vomiting. First because it takes too much milk and cannot digest it. Second/ because the milk is too thin/ watery/ moist/ and runny. Third because the milk is impure. And the baby will vomit due to these three causes especially/ when it has

*Coconut.

a moist sick stomach. And it should be helped thus/ give it a little to suckle/ then pay close attention to the vomit/ if it tastes like vinegar/ and it is white then take eight wheat corns' weight of frankincense/ and .xx. wheat corns' weight of dried rue/ make these things to a pulver and add them to rose syrup and give it to the baby. Or the wet-nurse should take roman caraway/ and chew it well/ and spread it in the baby's mouth/ or give it pomegranate syrup/ with pulverized mint. ¶Also another/ Take a dram of aloes wood/ one-half dram of mastic/ ten barley corns' weight of oak apple/ grind these things to a pulver/ temper it with rose syrup/ and with gallia muscata/ and give it to the baby before it nurses/ and lay this plaster on its stomach. Take equal amounts of mastic and sloe juice/ called accacia in Latin/ aloe epaticum/ oak apple/ frankincense/ and toasted bread/ grind these things and temper them with roses and with rose syrup/ and make a plaster on the baby's stomach. ¶Furthermore if the baby's vomit does not taste or smell like vinegar/ but rather has some other strong smell/ and the woman is pale/ but not completely white*/ then give the baby juice from unripe grapes/ or quince juice. ¶Also a plaster for this. Take barley flour/ and little green shoots from blackberry bushes/ and pomegranate rinds/ grind these things and temper them with rose water/ and lay this on its stomach. ¶And if the baby has a bad moist undigesting stomach/ then rub its stomach with rose water/ in which musk has been blended/ or with water from an herb called mirtus/ and give it a drink of quince juice with a little clove/ and sugar/ or one-third of a dram of gallia muscata/ with a little quince juice.

On Nightmares

¶Babies also have frightening dreams/ these usually come from overeating/ and are helped thus/ do not let it sleep with a

---

*The German reads "und die fraw nit gantz wyβ were/ besunder bleich far"; this may be a printer's error. An alternate interpretation would be "the vomit is pale/ but not white."

full stomach. And give it a little honey to lick/ so that it will digest what is in its stomach/ and push it down to the bowels. ¶Also give it daily one-seventh of an electuary called dyamuscus/ or dyapliris/ and tiriaca given with milk is especially good as Rhazes says.

Predisposition to Falling Sickness

¶Babies also get a sickness called the mother/ in Latin mater puerorum/ and it comes to them when they are nursing, and these are the symptoms. They cry a lot and become frightened in their sleep/ and do not sleep well/ and become hot/ and have stinking breath/ and such a sickness comes/ because the baby suckles more milk than it can digest/ help this baby as follows. Make the wet-nurse's milk good so that the baby can digest it. ¶Also give it one-sixth part of a dram of an electuary called dyapliris or dyamuscus daily/ and it is especially good to give it treacle stirred in milk.

A Rasping Breath

¶Babies are also stricken with a heavy/ narrow/ short breath when they sleep/ that is when they breathe they rasp/ and their breath pushes against them with a tone that can be noticeably heard. Help them as follows. Take well-powdered linseeds and mix them with well-clarified honey and spread it often in the baby's mouth. ¶Also if the baby does not have a high heat/ then take well-pulverized roman caraway/ and mix it with clarified honey and spread it in.

Protrusion of the Rectum

¶It also happens to babies that the rectum comes out/ and when that happens/ then take equal amounts of pomegranate rinds and an herb called mirtus/ acorn husks/ dried rose leaves/ burned hartshorn/ alum/ goat's hooves or shoes/ pomegranate blossoms/ and oak apple. Boil all these things well in water until the water receives the power of these things/ then bathe the baby in this water when it is lukewarm.

Tenasmon

¶Babies are also stricken with a sickness called tenasmon in Latin/ which is that the baby has the desire to pass stools/ and works hard and pushes greatly/ but achieves little or nothing/ and this usually comes from the cold, and is helped as follows. Take equal amounts of well-pulverized watercress seeds and roman caraway seeds/ and mix it with old cow's butter and give it to the baby to drink in cold water. ¶Also another/ Take turpentine and lay it on glowing coals/ and let the vapors from it go up into the baby's rectum. ¶Also another. Take scammony called colofonia in Latin lay it on an ember/ and let the vapor go into the baby's behind.

On Worms in the Rectum

¶When worms grow in the baby's rectum the size of cheese mites or smaller/ or when long worms grow in its body/ Then take witch grass water called gramen in Latin/ and give it to it in milk. ¶Also another/ Take one-third of a dram each of white coral/ shaved ivory/ burned hartshorn/ and iris that is violet root/ and five lots of white sugar/ and enough witch grass water/ have little plugs made out of this at the apothecary/ and give the baby two drams daily. ¶Also another Rhazes writes. Take roman caraway well pulverized with ox bile/ make a plaster out of it and lay it on the baby's navel. ¶Also olive oil given internally kills all the worms in the baby. ¶Also kill the small worms thus. Take cotton and make a little plug out of it/ moisten it in wormwood oil/ or rue oil/ or peach-stone oil/ or bitter almond oil/ and shove it in the baby's bottom. It is also good to bathe the baby in water in which peach leaves and wormwood have been boiled. ¶Also another. Make a salve with which you rub the baby's body near the worms. Take one-half lot each of wormwood and lupines/ and one lot each of the seed siler montan/ roman caraway/ black coriander called nigella in Latin/ lesser centaury called centaurea in Latin/ wormseeds/ and burned hartshorn/ grind these things fine and mix them with four lots each of wormwood oil and bitter almond oil/ and one lot of wax/ make a salve out of this and use it as described above. ¶Also a plaster against worms. Take two drams black coriander called nigella in Latin/ one dram each aloe/ red coral/ one-half lot each of wormwood/ mastic/ one and one-half lots of macerated coriander/ pulverize these things finely with six lots of rye flour/ and with one and one-half lots of lupines also powdered/ and a dram of saffron/ mix these with four lots of rue juice, and if you do not have the juice/ then take the same amount of wormwood oil/ and make a plaster out of it/ and lay it a hand's width on the baby's navel. ¶Also another plaster/ particularly for long worms/ Take four lots each of wormwood juice and ox bile/ two lots well pulverized colocynth/ make a plaster with a little rye flour/ and lay it warm on the baby's navel. ¶Also a bath for worms/ boil wormwood and oak apples in water/ and bathe the baby in it up to the navel.

When a Baby Becomes Sore and Chafed on Its Skin

¶Chafing of the baby on the skin/ of its legs and behind comes from the sharpness of the urine. And to counter the chafing take the herb mirtus well powdered and sprinkle it on. Or take iris/ red roses/ wild galangal/ or gum tragacanth/ or one or all well pulverized/ and sprinkle it on. ¶Also a salve for this/ Take .ii. lots of rose oil/ a dram of frankincense and melt them together/ and eight barley corns' weight of camphor/ and stir the camphor beforehand in rose water/ make a salve/ and smear the baby with it. ¶Furthermore a salve called ungentum album or ungentum de cerusa in Latin/ and a salve called ungentum rubeum/ are also good for this.

On Falling Sickness*

¶Furthermore babies are stricken with falling sickness/ and in two ways. First the baby is born with the sickness/ and it comes from coldness and bad fluids in the brain. Second the falling sickness comes from circumstances after the birth. If the baby has the disease by nature/ then keep it sound with food and drink which are warm and dry/ and the wet-nurse should do the same for herself. ¶Also if falling sickness comes to a baby in its infancy/ it does not leave a boy before .xxv. years/ or a girl until her menstruation comes for the first time. And if the sickness is not remedied quickly with medicines or by nature/ then the child be it boy or girl will not be able to become free of the sickness. If however the disease comes from circumstances after the birth/ then one should take care that the wet-nurse's milk is good and natural. For this it is necessary/ that you purge the wet-nurse's head with appropriate medicines and the wet-nurse should avoid all cold moist foods/ and should not feed the baby more than it can digest, and put castor oil/ costus oil/ or spurge oil in its nostrils/ and have it smell rue/ and the aromatic gum called asafetida in Latin. One should also hang peony seeds and roots gathered in a waning moon around the baby's neck, and if it is necessary/ give it treacle. ¶Also another/ Give the baby hare's rennet called coagulum leporis in Latin to drink in honey water/ and on the same day do not give it any milk. ¶Also hang on the baby's neck oak mistletoe which has been cut in March under a waning moon. ¶Also there are many more things which are good for this sickness which have been left out for the sake of brevity.

*Epilepsy.

When a Baby Is Too Thin and Gaunt

¶If the baby loses much weight so that there is nothing on it but skin and bone/ and it becomes very sick and weak/ then make a water bath for it in which the head and feet of a ram have been boiled/ and you should boil these in the water until the meat falls from the bones/ and you should bathe the baby in this bath frequently. And when you take it out of the bath/ you should dry it well and rub it with this salve/ take .iii. lots each of unrefined butter and violet oil or rose oil/ one and one-half lots of pig fat and one lot of white wax/ melt these things and make a salve/ smear the baby with this every day after its bath/ it will gain weight and become fat from this. ¶Also another salve. Take white wax/ and pig fat/ sheep tallow and unrefined butter/ Melt all these things over coals and sieve them through a cloth and use as above.

When a Baby Becomes Lame

And its limbs hang loose and dangle so that it cannot control its limbs and will not be able to walk at the proper time. If it is still nursing/ then give the wet-nurse medicines which warm and dry and also give her a lot of roasts/ and baked goods to eat/ and no milk fish or hard meat. She should also not mix wine with the water she drinks/ and before the wet-nurse nurses the baby she should bathe it/ and rub it with castoreum oil/ or chestnut oil. ¶Also give the baby a little of this electuary each day. Take a dram each of wild mint/ cinnamon sticks/ roman caraway/ dried rose leaves/ mastic/ fenugreek/ valerian/ ameos/ doronicum*/ zedoary/ cloves/ sandalwood/ and aloes wood/ and one-half dram of bisaz. Make these things into a powder and make an electuary out of it with a little clarified honey and give the baby one-half of one-half of a dram each day. ¶If the baby is lame in all its limbs/ then take two lots of wax and a dram of

*Leopard's bane.

well-ground spurge/ and enough olive oil and make a plaster out of it/ and lay it on the baby's spine.

Trembling of the Limbs

¶Furthermore if the baby gets a trembling in its limbs/ Then it is to be feared that it will become lame/ and stricken with falling sickness/ Help this baby as follows. Take rose oil/ and spikenard oil mixed together/ or another warm oil/ like laurel oil/ warm and rub the baby's spine with these well and also rub the limbs which tremble/ and if this is not enough then seek further advice from the doctors.

Stones in the Bladder

¶And if the baby has stones in its bladder/ or some other obstruction which blocks the urine. Then these are the signs/ the baby has burning urination and urinates frequently/ a little at a time with great pain/ and pushing/ and the urine is pale and clear/ and if it is a boy/ then his penis is stiff all the time. Help the baby as follows/ bathe it in warm water/ in which mallows/ althea/ linseeds/ and pellitory of the wall/ called paritaria in Latin have been boiled. Then give the baby something that gently drives and brings out its urine/ and when you lay the baby to sleep/ then rub the baby around the genitals with olive oil/ and give it blackberry tea in milk to drink. ¶Also another/ Take buck's blood/ and burned scorpion powder/ pulverize all of these/ and mix them with scorpion oil/ or white-lily oil/ and lay it on the baby's body above the genitals.

When the Baby Squints

¶Furthermore if the baby squints in one eye/ then place the rocker so that the baby sees the light directly opposite/ and not above it or next to it/ and if it squints or is cross-eyed on one side/ then turn the rocker so that the other side is against the light in the day/ and at night set a burning candle/ on the side where it does not squint/ so that it sees the light at all times/ equally on the side that does not squint during the day and also the night. Also hang near and for it beautiful pretty cloths of various color/ and especially those with a gold/ or green color/ so that its face is turned and pulled away from the squinting/ and inclined toward the other side/ and do this until the face is turned/ and even. And with that this little book is ended.

Table

Here in this little book there are many Latin words/ and this is because one cannot always bring this Latin into good German/ so that it would be understandable to women/ They should take refuge with the doctors and apothecaries/ who will give them sufficient instruction in all of this. In addition many of the herbs do not have one name in all of the German lands/ as for example absinthium in Latin/ is called wormwood [*wermut*] in Straβurg/ absinthe [*wygen*] in Frankfurt/ and wormwood [*elsen*] in Trier. For this reason here follows a table in which one can find the Latin and German &c.*

Latin	English
Aamidum	starch
Abrothanum	southernwood
Absinthium	wormwood/absinthe
Accacia†	sloe juice
Alipta muscata	an aromatic confection which they have at the apothecary
Aloe epaticum	a bitter juice called by this name [bitter aloes]
Aloes lignum	aloes wood
Althea	marshmallow/althea
Ambra	an aromatic thing which comes from a fish [ambergris]
Amigdalum amatum	bitter almonds

*Here, of course, in English translation. Names of herbs in brackets are editorial additions to clarify meaning. The list has also been put into strict alphabetical order.
†Acacia: "a kinde of thorne: also the iuice of the same fruit, in steede whereof men do use the iuice of sloes." (Thomas)

Latin	**English**
Amigdalum dulce	sweet almonds
Anetum	dill
Anisum	aniseed
Antera	the yellow seeds in roses
Anthimonium	antimony
Aristologia longa	birthwort (long)
Aristologia rotunda	birthwort (round)
Armoniacum	a gum called by this name [gum ar-moniac]
Arthanita	sowbread
Arthimesia	mugwort
Asafetida	devil's dung/ferula
Azarum	European snakeroot/hazelwort
Baccelauri	laurel/bayleaves/laurel berries
Balaustia	pomegranate flowers
Barotus	blind nettle/dead nettles with white-yellow flowers/"our lady's slippers"
Bdellim	a gum called by this name
Bitumen iudaicum	dry pitch of India
Bolus armenus	a red earth
Bothermarien	sowbread
Branca ursina	bear's foot/stinking hellebore
Bursa pastoris	shepherd's purse
Butyrum	butter/fat
Camedreos	germander
Camomila	camomile flowers
Camphora	camphor
Capillus veneris	maidenhair/rock fern
Cardamomum	cardamom
Carui	caraway
Cassia lignea	a bark called by this name [senna]
Castanea	chestnut
Castoreum	castoreum
Centaurea	European centaury/lesser centaury
Cerebrum leporis	hare's brain
Cerefolium	chervil
Ciminum	roman caraway
Cinamomum	cinnamon

Table   123

Latin	English
Ciperus	wild galangal
Citonia	quince
Coagulum hedi	kid's rennet
Coagulum leporis	hare's rennet
Colofonia	scammony
Coloquintida	colocynth
Consolida maior	wallwort/comfrey
Copule glandium	acorn husks
Corallus albus	white coral
Corallus rubeus	red coral
Coriandrum	coriander
Cornu cerui combustum	burned hartshorn
Costus amarus	a bitter herb called by this name [costus]
Cotum	cottonseed
Cristallus	crystals
Crocus	saffron
Cucurbita	pumpkin
Cycer	chickpeas
Doronicum	a root called by this name [leopard's bane]
Dragagantum	a white gum called by this name [gum tragacanth]
Dyptamus	dittany/fraxinella
Ebulus	dwarf elder
Edela arborea	ivy/that grows on trees
Elleborus albus	white hellebore/sneezewort
Elleborus niger	Christmas rose/black hellebore
Ematites	hematite (a stone)
Euforbium	a gum called by this name [spurge]
Extrematites vitis	the sour knobs on the grapevine
Farina molendini	flour dust
Farina ordei	barley flour
Fel thauri	ox bile
Fel vacce	cow bile
Fermentum	yeast/leaven
Ficus	figs

Latin	**English**
Filex	stone fern/male fern
Fimus accipitris	hawk dung
Fimus columbarum	pigeon dung
Flores rosarum	rose petals
Folia lauri	bay leaves
Folia persicorum	peach leaves
Folia rosarum vel	rose leaves
Furfur	groats/bran
Galanga	galanga/catarrh root
Galbanum	a smelly gum called by this name
Galla	oak apple/gall nut
Gallia muscata	an aromatic confection found at the apothecary [French musk]
Gariofili	cloves
Glans	acorn
Gramen	grass/couch grass
Grana iuniperi	juniper berries
Karabe	yellow amber
Lactuca	lettuce
Laudanum	an aromatic black gum [tincture of opium]
Licium	a juice called by this name
Macis	mace
Maiorana	marjoram
Malum granatum	pomegranate
Malva	mallows
Marrubium	horehound
Matricaria	feverfew/camomile
Menta	mint
Menta aquatica	water mint
Mercurialis	dog's mercury
Micleta	an electuary called by this name
Milium	millet seed
Millissa	balm/melissa
Mirra	a gum resin [myrrh]
Mirtilli	blueberry/bilberry
Mirtus	myrtle
Morabacci	blackberry

Table   125

Latin	English
Moracelsi	mulberry
Muscus	musk
Nasturcium	watercress
Nespilum	medlars
Nigella	black coriander
Nuclei persicorum	peach stone
Nux cipressi	cypress nut
Nux indica	coconut
Nux muscata	nutmeg
Oleum amigdalarum amararum	bitter almond oil
Oleum amigdalarum dulcium	sweet almond oil
Oleum anetinum	dill oil
Oleum camomillinum	camomile oil
Oleum costinum	oil of costus
Oleum de absinthio	absinthe oil/wormwood oil/ vermouth oil
Oleum de castoreo	castoreum oil
Oleum de euforbio	spurge oil
Oleum de keyri	yellow–clove blossom oil
Oleum de spica	spike lavender oil
Oleum laurinum	laurel oil
Oleum liliorum alborum	white-lily oil
Oleum mirtinum	myrtle oil
Oleum olivarum	olive oil
Oleum pulegi	pennyroyal oil
Oleum rosarum	rose oil
Oleum rutaceum	rue oil
Oleum violarum	violet oil
Oleum yrinum	blue-lily oil
Olibanum	frankincense/white incense
Opium	a juice made from poppy seeds
Oppoponacum	a gum called by this name
Ordeum excorticatum	peeled or shelled barley/crushed barley
Origanum	dittany
Papaver album	white poppyseeds

Latin	**English**
Paritaria	pellitory of the wall
Passule	raisin/grape
Pastinaca	parsnip
Penthafilon	cinquefoil
Peonia	peony root
Petrosilium	parsley
Pinguedo anatis	duck fat
Pinguedo anseris	goose fat
Pinguedo galline	chicken fat
Pix navalis	ship's pitch
Plantago maior	broad-leaved plantain
Plantago minor	lance-leaved plantain/ribwort
Policaria	an herb called by this name [fleabane]
Portulaca	purslane
Prassium	horehound
Proserpinata	knot grass
Psidia	pomegranate rinds
Pulegium	pennyroyal
Rasura de cornu capre	scraped from goat horn
Rasura eboris	ivory/scraped from elephant bone
Risum	rice
Rosmarinus	rosemary
Rubea tinctorum	"red" for dying — an herb/madder
Ruta	rue
Sambuccus	black elder
Sandalum rubeum	red sandalwood
Savina	savin
Se. bombicis	cotton seeds
Se. cucurbite	pumpkin seeds
Se. feniculi	fennel seeds
Se. lappacij acut	burdock seeds
Se. pionie	peony seeds
Serapinum	a smelly gum
Serpentinal	different plants with snake-like roots
Serpillum	wild thyme/wild pennyroyal

Table   127

Latin	English
Solatrum	nightshade
Sorbe	sorb-service berries
Spodium	ivory black/burned elephant bone
Staphisagria	stavesacre/larkspur/lousewort
Stercus muris	nutmeg
Succus citomorum	quince juice
Succus liquiricie	licorice juice
Sumach	a sour red fruit [sumac]
Tamariscus	tamarisc
Tapsus barbatus	mullein
Tormentilla	tormentil/shepherd's knot
Valeriana	valerian
Virga pastoris	shepherd's rod/Fuller's thistle/ teazel
Vuapassa	big raisin/grape
Wullina	mullein/king's candle
Xiloaloes	aloe
Xilocaracta	carob bean
Yreos	iris root
Zedoaria	zedoary
Zuccarum	sugar
Zuccarum pendiarum	sugar penids

BIBLIOGRAPHY

Arms, Suzanne. *Immaculate Deception: A New Look at Women and Childbirth in America.* Boston: Houghton Mifflin, 1975.

Aveling, J.H. *English Midwives: Their History and Prospects.* 1872. Reprint. London: Hugh K. Elliot, 1967.

Avicenna. *The General Principles of Avicenna's Canon of Medicine.* Translated by Mazhar H. Shah. Karachi, Pakistan: Naveed Clinic, 1966.

Baas, Karl. "Dr. Eucharius Rösslin: Arzt zu Worms im 16. Jahrhundert." *Vom Rhein: Monatsschrift des Altertumsvereins für die Stadt Worms.* Vol. 2 (1903): 38–40.

──────. *Eucharius Rösslins Lebensgang.* Separatabdruck aus dem *Archiv für Geschichte der Medizin.* Edited by Karl Sudhoff. Volume 1, number 6. Leipzig: Johann Ambrosius Barthe, 1908.

──────. "Zur Lebensgeschichte Rösslins." *Vom Rhein: Monatsschrift des Altertumsvereins für die Stadt Worms.* Vol. 4 (1905): 70–71.

Biographisches Lexikon der hervorragenden Ärzte aller Zeiten und Völker. Edited by August Hirsch. Volume 4, 2d edition. Berlin: Urban, 1932.

Boesch, Hans. *Kinderleben in der deutschen Vergangenheit.* Monographien zur deutschen Kulturgeschichte. Volume 5. Leipzig, 1900.

Brian, Peter. *Galen on Bloodletting.* Cambridge: Cambridge University Press, 1986.

Callaway, Helen. "'The Most Essentially Female Function of All': Giving Birth." In *Defining Females,* pp. 163–86. Edited by Shirley Ardener. London: Croom Helm, in association with the Oxford University Women's Studies Committee, 1978.

Chamberlain, Mary. *Old Wives' Tales: Their History, Remedies and Spells.* London: Virago, 1981.

Cianfrani, Theodore. *A Short History of Obstetrics and Gynecology.* Springfield, Ill.: Charles C. Thomas, 1960.

Cooke, Cynthia W. and Susan Dworkin. *The Ms. Guide to a Woman's Health.* Garden City, N.Y.: Anchor, 1979.

Culpepper, Nicholas. *Pharmacopoeia Londinensis.* By Peter Cole, 1659.

Cutter, Irving, and Henry Viets. *A Short History of Midwifery.* Philadelphia: W. B. Saunders, 1964.

Diepgen, Paul. *Frau und Frauenheilkunde in der Kultur des Mittelalters.* Stuttgart: Georg Thieme, 1963.

Donegan, Jane. *Women and Men Midwives.* Westport, Conn.: Greenwood, 1978.

Donnison, Jean. *Midwives and Medical Men: A History of Interprofessional Rivalries and Women's Rights.* New York: Schocken Books, 1977.

Eccles, Audrey. *Obstetrics and Gynecology in Tudor and Stuart England.* Kent, Ohio: Kent State University Press, 1982.

Ehrenreich, Barbara, and Deirdre English. *Witches, Midwives and Nurses: A History of Women Healers.* Old Westbury, N.Y.: Feminist Press, 1973.

Engelsing, Rolf. *Analphabetentum und Lektüre: zur Sozialgeschichte des Lesens in Deutschland zwischen feudaler und industrieller Gesellschaft.* Stuttgart: J. B. Metzler, 1973.

Fasbender, H. *Geschichte der Geburtshülfe.* Jena: Gustav Fischer, 1906.

Fischer, Alfons. *Geschichte des deutschen Gesundheitswesens.* Hrsgbn. von der Arbeitsgemeinschaft sozialhygienischer Reichsfachverbande. 2 volumes. Berlin: Kommissionsverlag F. A. Herbig, 1933.

Forbes, Thomas. *The Midwife and the Witch.* New Haven, Conn.: Yale University Press, 1966.

————. "Regulation of English Midwives in the 16th and 17th Centuries." *Medical History* 8. (1964): 235–44.

Götze, Alfred. *Frühneuhochdeutsches Glossar.* Bonn: A. Marcus and E. Webers, 1912.

Graham, Harvey. *Eternal Eve.* New York: Doubleday, 1951.

Haggard, Howard W. *Devils, Drugs, and Doctors.* New York: Harper and Row, 1929.

Hippocrates. *The Aphorisms of Hippocrates.* Translated by Elias Marks. New York: Collins, 1817.

Hughes, Muriel Joy. *Women Healers in Medieval Life and Literature.* New York: King's Crown, 1943.

Illich, Ivan. *Gender.* New York: Pantheon, 1982.

Ingerslev, E. "Rösslin's 'Rosegarten': Its Relation to the Past (the Muscio Manuscripts and Soranos), Particularly with Regard to Podalic Version." *Journal of Obstetrics and Gynaecology of the British Empire* 15, no. 1 (January 1909): 1–92.

Jameson, Edwin. *Gynecology and Obstetrics.* New York: Hafner, 1962.

Jonas, Richard. *The Byrth of Mankynde.* Imprinted in London, by T.R., 1540.

Kallmorgen, Dr. Wilhelm. *Siebenhundert Jahre Heilkunde in Frankfurt am Main.* Frankfurt am Main: Moritz Diesterweg, 1936.

Klein, Gustav, ed. *Eucharius Rösslins "Rosengarten."* In *Alte Meister der Medizin and Naturkunde.* Munich: Carl Kuhn, 1910.

Knefelkamp, Ulrich. *Das Gesundheits- und Fürsorgewesen der Stadt Freiburg im Breisgau im Mittelalter.* Freiburg im Breisgau: Herder Buchhandlung, 1981.

Needham, Joseph. *A History of Embryology.* New York: Abelard Schumann, 1959.

Ozment, Steven. *When Fathers Ruled: Family Life in Reformation Europe.* Cambridge, Mass.: Harvard University Press, 1983.

Radcliffe, Walter. *Milestones in Midwifery.* Bristol, England: John Wright and Sons, 1967.

Rösslin, Eucharius. *Der Swangern frawen und he bammen roszgarten.* In *Alte Meister der Medizin und Naturkunde.* Munich: Carl Kuhn, 1910.

Rothman, Barbara Katz. *In Labor: Women and Power in the Birthplace.* New York: W. W. Norton, 1982.

Rowland, Beryl. *Medieval Woman's Guide to Health.* Kent, Ohio: Kent State University Press, 1981.

Scherzer, Ricarda. *Hebammen: Weise Frauen oder Technikerinnen? Zum Wandel eines Berufsbildes.* Frankfurt am Main: Inst. für Kulturanthropologie und Europäische Ethnologie, 1988.

Semmelweis, Ignaz. *The Etiology, Concept, and Prophylaxis of Childbed Fever.* Translated by K. Codell Carter. Wisconsin Publications in the History of Science and Medicine, no. 2. Madison: University of Wisconsin Press, 1983.

Sharp, Jane. *The Midwives Book.* 1671. Reprint. New York: Garland, 1985.

Shorter, Edward. *A History of Women's Bodies.* New York: Basic Books, 1982.

Siebold, Casper Jacob von. *Versuch einer Geschichte der Geburtshülfe.* Tübingen: Franz Pietzcker, 1901.

Soranus. *Soranus' Gynecology.* Translated by Owsei Temkin. Baltimore: Johns Hopkins University Press, 1956.

Strauss, Gerald. "Techniques of Indoctrination: The German Reformation." In *Literacy and Social Development in the West: A Reader,* pp. 96–104. Edited by Harvey J. Graff. New York: Cambridge University Press, 1981.

Stürzbecher, Manfred. "The Physici in German-Speaking Countries from the Middle Ages to the Enlightenment." In *The Town and State Physician in Europe from the Middle Ages to the Enlightenment,* pp. 123–29. Edited by Andrew W. Russell. Wolfenbüttel: Herzog August Bibliothek, 1981.

Thomas, Thomas. *Dictionarium Linguae Latinae et Anglicanae.* [1587]. Menston, England: Scolar, 1972.

Trotula of Salerno. *The Diseases of Women.* Translation of *Passionibus Mulierum Curandorum.* Translated by Elizabeth Mason-Hohl. Los Angeles: Ward-Ritchie, 1940.

Ungar, Helga. "Vorreden deutscher Sachliteratur des Mittelalters als Ausdruck literarischen Bewußtseins." In *Werk Typ Situation: Studien zu poetologischen Bedingungen in der älteren deutschen Literatur,* pp. 217–51. Edited by Ingeborg Glier. Stuttgart: J. B. Metzler, 1969.

Wiesner, Merry E. "Early Modern Midwifery: A Case Study." *International Journal of Women's Studies.* 6, no. 1 (January/February 1983): 26–43.

_____. *Working Women in Renaissance Germany.* New Brunswick, N.J.: Rutgers University Press, 1986.

INDEX